BALANCE
YOUR HE

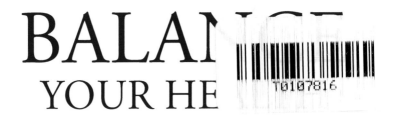

COMBINING CONVENTIONAL
AND NATURAL MEDICINE

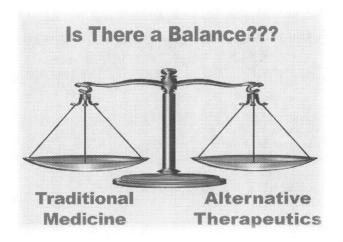

Is There a Balance???

Traditional Medicine

Alternative Therapeutics

Richard Sollazzo, MD
With Ronni Sollazzo, MD

iUniverse LLC
Bloomington

Balance Your Health
Combining Conventional and Natural Medicine

iUniverse books may be ordered through booksellers or by contacting:

iUniverse LLC
1663 Liberty Drive
Bloomington, IN 47403
www.iuniverse.com
1-800-Authors (1-800-288-4677)

ISBN: 978-1-4697-6519-8 (sc)
ISBN: 978-1-4697-6520-4 (hc)
ISBN: 978-1-4697-6521-1 (e)

Library of Congress Control Number: 2013908158

Printed in the United States of America

iUniverse rev. date: 11/23/2013

BALANCE
YOUR HEALTH

CONTENTS

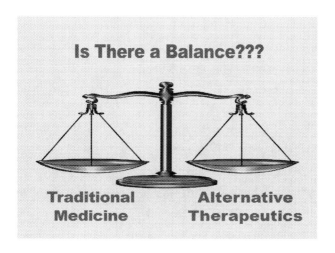

Is There a Balance???

Traditional Medicine   Alternative Therapeutics

CHAPTER 1

THE FIRST WAKE-UP CALL

When I was in medical school, I lost contact with several friends and acquaintances. I returned to New York and attempted to contact a close friend who was, like me, a health advocate. She was a vegetarian, took vitamin supplements, and was into "spiritual things." I was taken aback when I was told she had died of breast cancer.

I investigated what had happened to her. Her physician diagnosed her with clinical Stage I cancer of the left breast (localized tumor, less than two centimeters without spread to lymph nodes or other body areas). She was told by both her oncologists that if she followed a treatment plan consisting of surgery, possibly radiation therapy, and chemotherapy, she would have, most likely, a 95–97 percent cure rate. Her exact treatment plan would be dependent upon the results of the initial biopsy (e.g., breast tumor margins: whether clear or not of cancer cells; whether the cells were estrogen or progesterone positive or negative; and how many lymph nodes have cancer within them).

She was also told that without the treatment, she would likely die within two years. Since she strongly opposed chemotherapy and radiation, her oncologist strongly urged her to have, at the very least, the breast tumor removed and then consider alternative therapies. After careful consideration, she refused chemo, radiation, and the excisional biopsy of the breast mass. She decided to follow a course of alternative treatments exclusively. She fasted; took various herbs, vitamins, enzymes, and coffee enemas; and went abroad for what I was told was "injection therapy" (B17, other vitamins, and enzymes).

While maintaining her chosen treatment plan, her health deteriorated. She did not follow up with a medical doctor to see if her treatments were working. Approximately sixteen months after her diagnosis was made, she was doing poorly. She was severely weak and slept eleven to twelve hours per day. She developed severe headaches and vomited profusely. She had deteriorated to the point where her daughter found her lying in bed soaked in urine and feces.

She was taken by ambulance to the hospital where she was diagnosed with end-stage cancer. At this point in her disease, conventional curative treatment for the cancer could no longer be offered. All the doctors could do was care for her basic needs and provide adequate pain relief.

After my friend's death, I had lengthy discussions with her daughter so that I could come to terms with her mother's choices. After all, I was in medical school and was learning how to aggressively combat disease. She felt that her mother had "connected to natural living and alternative treatments" the majority of her life, as though it had been her religion. It had been her personal and philosophical decision and her right to choose what treatments she would utilize.

It is everyone's right to choose whatever medical and/or alternative therapies he or she would like. Hopefully, that decision is based on achieving the highest possible quality of life and prolonging survival in an educated, balanced, realistic, and clear-minded approach.

I discussed this case with four other complementary/integrative practitioners and two traditional oncologists who *all believed she should have had the breast cancer removed with lymph node dissection*, with further treatment based on these findings.

It should be mentioned that some feel if Mr. Steven Jobs had had surgery early on, he may have had a much better survival outcome. Why let the cancer cells have a chance to grow and travel to other parts of the body? Mr. Jobs felt surgery was too invasive—a decision he later regretted—and said, "I didn't want my body to be opened . . . I didn't want to be violated that way" (Henry Blodget, "Steve Jobs Refused Early Surgery for His Pancreatic Cancer, Isaacson Says—A Decision He Later Regretted," *Business Insider*, access date," http://articles. businessinsider.com/2011-10-20/tech/30301240_1_pancreatic-cancer-walter-isaacson-alternativetherapies). *Treating localized cancer quickly as possible with surgery can be lifesaving!* This statement cannot be overemphasized!

I have seen well more than a hundred patients *die needlessly* because they simply did not remove the cancer when it was localized and curable! If you or somebody you know is in a similar situation, do not let this be the outcome! Some feel cancer has a mind of its own and has no mercy. *Remove it from your body before it takes it over and you cannot be cured! You have to fight fire with fire!*

Of course there are exceptions. For example, it may be difficult to treat a low-grade, early-stage prostate cancer in an elderly patient with comorbidities (other diseases). In this case, the risks of surgery outweigh the possible benefits.

I tried to reconcile how my friend's illness tied into my own beliefs about health care. I had spent my life giving great value to natural therapeutics, yet here I was entrenched in a conventional medical training program, which at that time did not value these ideas. Differences between conventional medicine and alternative treatments are easily recognized and will be discussed in detail in later chapters. However, there are many similarities, such as agreement about the importance of exercise, nutrition, vitamins, and risk-factor modification (such as stopping smoking, eliminating obesity).

What has guided me through the rest of my medical career is the realization that there does not have to be a choice as to which approach to take. Medical care and treatment should be a *balance* of these two approaches. There shouldn't be a tug of war between these two systems of health care.

When one only uses "unproven"—scientifically speaking—methods of health care, we call this alternative, Eastern, or natural medicine.

Utilizing drugs, surgery, chemotherapy, and radiation is referred to as contemporary, traditional, customary, conventional, allopathic, Western, standard of care, or evidence-based medicine.

When one combines alternative and customary approaches, it is often referred to as complementary, integrative, or holistic medicine.

They should work in harmony to treat an illness and increase *health span* and *life span*. It is also extremely important to find and treat the cause, not the symptom, of an illness.

Always remember: *the cure is in the cause!*

LEVELS OF MEDICAL/HEALTH CARE

1. **Treating the symptom: headaches are not due to a deficiency of aspirin or pain reliever. There likely is an underlying cause. Headaches can be caused by stress, neck and head injuries, tumors in the brain, hypertension, and other disorders that should be ruled out.**

If your dog bites you, the cure is not only treating the dog bite but also the dog!

2. **Treating the *cause* of the symptom or illness.**

I have found that for physiological reasons, the cure is often in the cause. Finding the true cause for a symptom or overt illness will result in a true and lasting cure. Sometimes it is not possible to find the cause, even when using traditional and alternative medicine, since we do not know the cause of every symptom or overt disease that exists.

3. **Teaching the masses how to prevent illness and disease, improve health, and extend life span.**

An ounce of prevention is worth more than a pound of cure!

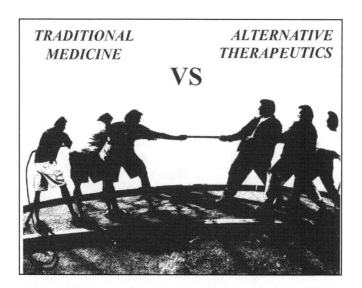

This book will present my approach to health care in my practice and in my life. Both customary and alternative medicine offer several beneficial and lifesaving diagnostic and therapeutic approaches. We will learn when and how to use each in a balanced, common sense, user-friendly, safe, and effective fashion for optimal results.

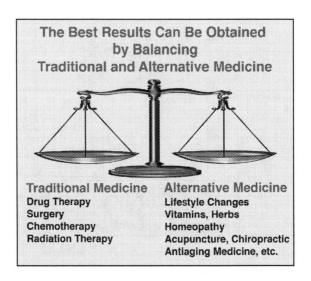

The Best Results Can Be Obtained
by Balancing
Traditional and Alternative Medicine

Traditional Medicine	Alternative Medicine
Drug Therapy	Lifestyle Changes
Surgery	Vitamins, Herbs
Chemotherapy	Homeopathy
Radiation Therapy	Acupuncture, Chiropractic
	Antiaging Medicine, etc.

CHAPTER 2

TRENDS IN MEDICAL PRACTICE

The part can never be well unless the whole is well.

—Plato

Medicine is the art of maintaining and restoring human health by studying, diagnosing, and treating disease with the ultimate goal of averting death. The diagnostic tools utilized can be lifesaving. Most treatments used are medication, surgery, and radiation. A healthy lifestyle is now emphasized by mainstream medicine.

One would have to agree that if your heart stops beating, or you're having an acute heart attack, seizure, stroke, or allergic reaction, traditional emergency medicine and not alternative would be the way to go. In such acute emergency situations, allopathic (traditional) medicine alone would be indicated and lifesaving. Vitamins, herbs, acupuncture, chiropractic, and other natural methods would not be able to rapidly stop such acute life-threatening medical situations; therefore they would not be applicable.

I have said, 'If you need a shovel,
one thousand pitchforks will not help!'

Early medical practice used natural resources, such as plants, animal parts, and minerals, in addition to religious and magical resources. The great school of Hippocrates in ancient Greece developed the theory of the four humors. It was felt that there were four substances in the human body: blood, phlegm, yellow bile, and black bile. Each substance was supposed to have attributes, and the four humors were supposed to be kept in balance. The main aim of the doctors was to create a balance of the humors in the body. Often, their methods were based on changes in diet.

Ancient Chinese medicine believed there were two forces that dominated the world: yin and yang. Their balance was necessary for health. The concept of balancing different forces to create health and longevity has been promulgated for many years and in many different cultures.

The goal of this book is to find a balance between conventional and alternative medicines in such as way as to use the best of both worlds to treat disease and create the longest possible disease-free life. *Thomas Edison said, 'The doctor of the future will no longer treat the human frame with drugs, but rather will cure and prevent disease with nutrition.'*

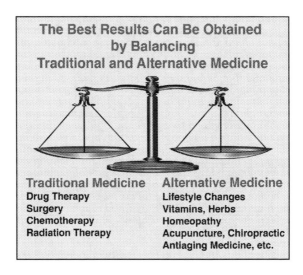

Alternative medicine emphasizes that when the body is at a high level of health it is less prone to overt disease. Dis-ease is considered the "lack of ease." Everyone has experienced a time when he or she was under a lot stress, not sleeping enough, not exercising, or eating poorly. When in this situation, you feel tired, cannot perform optimally, look tired (actually look and feel older), feel increased aches and pains, and are prone to illness.

Some feel that if a person lives this way for an extended period of time, he or she will increase his or her chances of getting an overt disease, including autoimmune diseases, cancers, and heart disease. All forms of medicine try to reduce the incidence of diseases.

Alternative medicine emphasizes the need to *treat the whole person*. Lifestyle is a key component when treating the whole person. This usually treats the cause of illness or prevents it. Lifestyle is explained in detail later in this book.

I have been treating a forty-four-year-old female doctor for several years. Her major complaint for years has been tiredness and body aches. I thought it was a simple fix, since she only slept two to three hours per night! No matter how I pleaded with her to get more sleep, she refused. As time passed, her joint pain continued to get worse.

She went to a rheumatologist, who performed several blood tests for multiple rheumatologic diseases. All tests were negative. She was diagnosed with a sero-negative rheumatologic disease (blood tests for specific diseases that could cause such symptoms were negative, but she is classified as having an underlying nonspecified rheumatological disease). She was placed on a medicine that had several possible serious side effects, including increased cancer risk. The medicine helped her joint pain.

She continued the medicine for about eight months until she broke her arm. She was unable to work and was sleeping a lot more. She also stopped taking the medication. After more than four months, she called me and said I'd been right, that her joint pain was totally gone because she was sleeping more. She finally realized the lack of sleep was causing her joint pain all along.

Ten months elapsed and she was still off the medicine and pain free! This should be a no-brainer, but too many times lifestyle choices are not given nearly the importance they should! You can enjoy a healthy lifestyle.

Evidence-based medicine refers to the establishment of the most effective methods of practice using scientific methods and well-controlled statistical studies by scientists. Conventional medicine practitioners typically use treatments that have been approved and recommended by the medical community. Statistical studies can take years to prove the safety and efficacy of a given treatment that conventional medicine may utilize. Such studies are needed to scientifically determine if a diagnostic tool and/or a treatment plan is truly beneficial.

Most would say that regular exercise is a health-promoting and life-extending habit. A March 12, 2012, article titled "Total Daily Physical Activity and Longevity in Old Age" in the *Archives of Internal Medicine* stated, "An objective measure of the total daily activity, including both exercise and nonexercise physical activity, is associated with longevity in the community-dwelling older persons."

It was obvious by both the general population and physicians that smoking was not good for one's health. However, it took *many years for the medical community to scientifically state that it was detrimental for one's health.* Now it is well known to be the most common cause of lung cancer. It is also known to cause other forms of cancers, as well as heart and lung diseases.

In some situations, such as a cancer that does not have an effective treatment program available, a patient cannot wait for such a study to be completed. If the alternative and standard medical treatment and/or diagnostic tool does not conflict with each other, then it would make sense to utilize both methods in a situation such as this. It would be the hope that they would complement and enhance each other. This could be in regard to enhancing treatment outcome and/or decreasing side effects.

There are exceptions. Some cancer treatments are utilized in mainstream medicine before they have been fully studied due to time constraints. As many cancers are aggressive and can cause rapid death, the time it would take to have a drug thoroughly studied and approved, sometimes many years, would mean that a possibly beneficial drug would not be available to many people who are sick now. Patients taking such experimental drugs must sign legal medical release forms indicating they are aware of the risks involved. This is called "treatment by compassionate consent."

What else can a conventional doctor do when there aren't solid clinical studies available? They can seek out what is called level IIIC recommendations ("opinions of respected authorities, based on clinical experience, descriptive studies"). This is advice from experienced phyisicans that can be utilized for situations where there aren't formal studies available.

It has taken years for people to realize what most would consider "no-brainers," such as the importance of exercise, eating a balanced diet, and proper sleep/rest in promoting optimal health. Yet it has taken years to prove the importance of these things through medical studies. Medicine and science must undergo such studies to ensure they are perceived as scientific fact and not "science fiction."

Complementary and antiaging medicine typically use alternative treatment plans that are not yet proven by statistically well-controlled studies, yet they are often effective and safe treatments. For example, male menopause, also called andropause, is a patient who has a below-normal testosterone level. Alternative medicine has utilized testosterone replacement therapy for many years. This met with resistance, just as anything new typically does. Testosterone replacement therapy has finally become mainstream medicine. Pharmaceutical companies have recently capitalized on this and now manufacture costly testosterone medications. Advertisements for testosterone preparations can now be seen on television.

Alternative medicine has recognized the need for testing and treating low testosterone in men *and women* for many years! Unfortunately, as with many other important health discoveries utilized by alternative medicine, credit was not given to these forward-thinking clinicians.

It has been said that you can judge the greatness of an inventor or an outside-the-box thinker by the number of arrows in his or her back. Most change comes with ridicule and resistance. I heard a talk given by the man who invented the MRI. He not only expected resistance, he thrived on it. He said it accelerated his drive to complete the invention!

The saying "If we are all thinking the same, someone isn't thinking" applies to "thinking outside the box" and trying to find new cures. Yet most are resistant to change. *Without change, there isn't progress!* New treatments should be utilized in a safe, scientific fashion in order to validate their efficacy.

Holistic, integrative, complementary, and antiaging medicines typically use alternative treatment plans that are not yet proven by statistically well-controlled studies. Yet they are often successful in their impact on patients' health. More specifically, alternative doctors have been saying for years that exercise is good for cardiovascular health. It took several years for mainstream medicine to agree with this obvious finding. Many studies have proven the health benefits of exercise.

Mainstream medicine, for the most part, requires statistical evidence-based studies before endorsing the use of a new diagnostic tool or a treatment. *This is needed to ensure that treatments are truly effective, and that the benefits outweigh the side effects.*

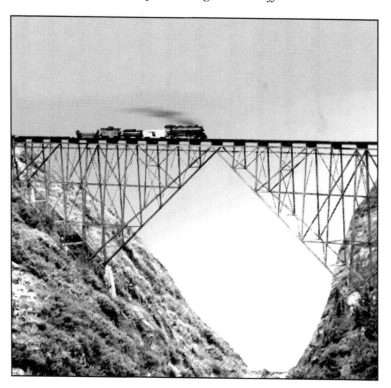

In conventional medicine, treatment is primarily aimed at the disease state. Traditional medicine also recommends early detection of disease via colonoscopies, imaging studies, blood and stress tests, and other diagnostic tools.

Holistic medicine utilizes therapies that attempt to treat the patient as a whole person, taking into account the individual's overall physical, mental, spiritual, and emotional well-being. Many alternative or natural therapies offer a holistic approach, but this is not always consistently the case. In my practice, I try to think outside, through, and around the box by cross-linking many forms of medical and alternative approaches for the best possible results. There are several reasons most physicians do not do this.

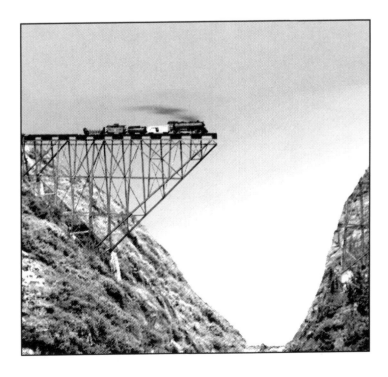

Each week, hundreds of medical discoveries are published in internationally recognized scientific and medical journals. Not all of these lifesaving and disease-preventing findings are made available to patients.

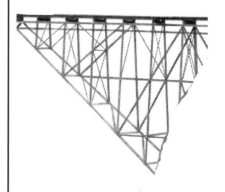

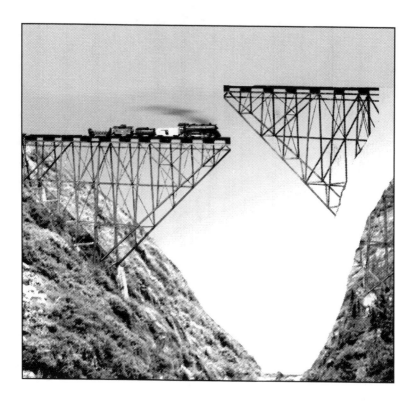

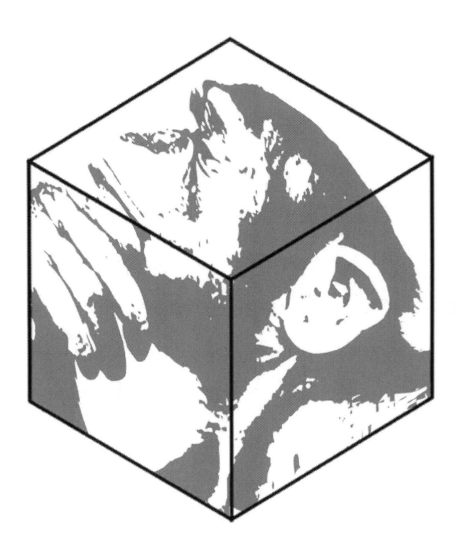

Medical triumph has involved thinking outside the box to find cures for disease and to find ways to increase our life span and improve our quality of life.

CHAPTER 3
ALTERNATIVE MEDICINE

Alternative treatments, for the most part, are considered unproven and are generally not medically accepted by mainstream medicine. They are not discussed in mainstream literature. Therefore, the majority of medical doctors do not know of many alternative approaches, never mind utilize them.

Unfortunately, scientific studies can take many years to obtain final results. Even more unfortunate is that there usually isn't funding available to test alternative treatments. *If a product is not patentable, pharmaceutical and other large businesses tend to not put money into research.* There is a saying in business: if there's no patent, there's no incentive. Hence the effectiveness of a product will not be scientifically established. In spite of this, a large portion of the public utilizes alternative treatments.

Alternative medicine should have statistical studies performed to scientifically move forward and stop the close-minded dinosaurs from trampling them.

An article titled "Unconventional Medicine in the United States: Prevalence, Costs, and Patterns of Use," published in the *New England Journal of Medicine* (328:246–52,1993) pointed out that in the early 1990s, the public visited more complementary and alternative practitioners than all primary care medical physicians.

An article published in the *American Journal of Hematology/ Oncology*, titled "Multidisciplinary Therapy: Integrated Medicine in Cancer Care" (October 2007, 552), stated that "as many as 80 percent of patients undergoing conventional treatment for cancer also use 'complementary' or 'alternative' care." Furthermore, it is stated that this trend continued throughout the '90s, and this number is anticipated to rise.

In a 2007 interview, the director of the National Center of Complementary and Alternative Medicine (NCCAM), Josephine Briggs, agreed that 38 percent of the population utilizes alternative medicine (http://nccam.nih.gov/ news/ multimedia/video/briggsvideo.htm).

Americans spend approximately one-third as much out-of-pocket money for over-the-counter supplements as prescription drugs. The cost of alternative medicine (patient visits, supplements, and other products utilized) is estimated at $34 billion per year. Please see WebMD for more details on this subject.

In fact, some consider "alternative" medicine not "alternative" at all. In an article titled "Alternative Medicine is Becoming Mainstream," written by Tammy Worth and published in the *Los Angeles Times* (November 2009, 3–4), discuses in detail that alternative may actually be considered mainstream medicine.

Drs. Deepak Chopra, Dean Ornish, Roy Rustum, and Andrew Weil have all written articles regarding "alternative" medicine becoming mainstream.

Until recently, antiaging/longevity medicine has been considered alternative medicine. According to *Time* magazine's twenty-two-page cover story, "Health Checkup: How to Live 100 Years," published in their February 22, 2010, issue, antiaging/longevity medicine has become mainstream. Many concepts and treatments that were considered alternative medicine are now accepted and utilized in customary medicine.

Most people want longer and healthier lives. However, not all are willing to take the appropriate steps necessary to take advantage of this field of medicine. A good example of this is exercising. I tell my patients jokingly that exercise is the hardest vitamin pill to swallow. If you want something, you have to do something, and health is no exception!

Some examples of what has been considered alternative therapies include:

Acupuncture

- A procedure used in or adapted from Chinese medical practice in which specific body areas are pierced with fine needles for therapeutic purposes (to treat illness alone or with other modalities of therapy and for general health) or to relieve pain or produce regional anesthesia.

Ayurveda Medicine

- An ancient system of medicine derived from the Hindu tradition in India. Among the treatments in Ayurveda is an internal purification via Shodan cleansing, depending on body type. Five cleansing methods are used, which include fomentation-sweating treatment to release toxins. Various colon-cleansing techniques such as enemas may be used.

Homeopathy

- A system for treating disease based on the administration of minute doses of a drug that in much greater amounts produces symptoms in healthy individuals similar to those of the disease itself.

In-depth discussions of these modalities are beyond the scope of this book, but it serves to illustrate that there are many treatment options available. While perusing this list, however, one can notice that many of the practices listed have common ground with conventional medicine. Please see *Mosby's Dictionary of Complementary & Alternative Medicine,* edited By Wayne B. Jonas, and the American College for Advancement in Medicine (ACAM) for more information on alternative therapies.

Throughout the book, I will discuss actual case studies describing specific disease states and how patients can be treated in a synergistic and additive fashion by combining the philosophies of conventional and alternative medicine with the ultimate shared goal of increasing health span and life span. This is perhaps the crux of the book: that the successful combination of these therapies will promote ultimate good health and well-being.

Integrative medicine not only emphasizes the physician-patient relationship, it focuses on the least invasive and least toxic methods to promote health by integrating allopathic (conventional) with alternative therapies. As you will see, integrative medicine looks at patients and diseases with a broad lens.

CHAPTER 4

THE PATIENT IN THE DOCTOR'S OFFICE

Medicine, for many centuries, has focused on the patient's symptoms. During an office visit, patients are asked many questions in what is called "the review of systems." Typical questions, for example, focus on the presence or absence of chest pain; difficulty breathing; excessive thirst or urination (which may indicate diabetes); pain or swelling of the joints; abdominal discomfort; change of appetite; etc.

Risk factors for disease are assessed, such as family history of heart disease, cancer, or asthma, and whether the patient has ever been told he or she has high cholesterol or high blood pressure. These are disease-oriented questions. They do not necessarily take into account the patient's lifestyle and how this could modify or affect a disease.

More recent trends in conventional and alternative medicine have concentrated on the patient as a whole, not just as a model for a disease state, and have also established the true importance of preventive medicine in prolonging life span and health span. The focus should not just be on sickness but also on *keeping a well person well. An ounce of prevention is worth more than a pound of cure.*

Early detection of disease is recommended by conventional medicine. This can be exemplified in conventional medicine by screening procedures such as colonoscopies, blood tests, and mammograms. These and other conventional tests can be lifesaving.

Finally, emphasis is placed on not just "treating the snakebites" but also on "killing the snake"! A healthy lifestyle may prevent disease and prolong a healthy life span. *Not getting a disease is even better than early detection of it.*

One of history's greatest inventors and thinkers, Thomas Edison, said, "The doctor of the future will no longer treat the human frame with drugs, but rather will cure and prevent disease with nutrition."

Alternative-medicine practitioners advocate extensive blood testing for hormone deficiencies, inflammation, viruses, and for heavy metals to prevent the development of disease and to promote a sense of health and well-being. Clearly it would be better to *prevent disease* in the first place than to treat it once it develops. While this may appear to be a bit simplistic and obvious, it cannot be overemphasized. Unfortunately, if you develop an overt disease such as a deadly cancer (advanced lung, esophageal, pancreatic, breast), *lifestyle* changes in and of themselves usually will not result in a cure. This is why it is so important to maintain a healthy lifestyle, so that you might not develop overt disease.

A healthy lifestyle should include abstaining from smoking, drinking alcohol, and drugs. Also, regular exercise, eating healthy (organic foods if possible), drinking eight to ten glasses of distilled water a day, sleeping approximately eight hours a day, maintaining healthy relations with friends and family, controlling stress, and enjoying a positive attitude attribute to good health and longevity. Maintaining a high level of health will reduce your chances of developing overt disease and will help lengthen your life span and increase vitality, productivity, and enjoyment of life.

Several mainstream medical journals have published statistically controlled studies revealing the many benefits of a healthy lifestyle. In fact, the American Medical Association's *Archives of Internal Medicine,* in their January 25, 2010, issue, cited numerous healthy lifestyle articles. The articles included ways to improve diet and increase exercise.

Exercise was found to help improve bone density, cognition, weight control, overall longevity in women age seventy or older, and increase quality of life in deconditioned institutionalized elderly persons. This study, although performed on females, is felt to also apply to males. There were other articles extolling the benefits of a healthy diet and weight loss. In fact, all the articles in this issue were about the benefits of exercise and diet (http://archinte.ama-assn.org/content/vol170/issue2/index.dtl)!

What do I mean by a healthy lifestyle? From a medical point-of-view, of course, this would include regular medical checkups, blood tests, other diagnostic and screening tests, and utilizing various integrative forms of medicine. What else should this include? A healthy diet and exercise are crucial. A positive attitude about life, healthy relationships with family and friends, security in the work place, and financial security all contribute to emotional and physical well-being.

Your doctor may ask whether you are sleeping well at night. If you sleep poorly or not enough, you wake up feeling ill, achy, irritable, and unable to concentrate, and even your physical appearance will be affected. People tend to look older if they haven't been sleeping properly.

My many long years of medical training have made me an expert on sleep deprivation and its consequences! If you have significant and consistent trouble sleeping, you should consult your practitioner, as there may be medical causes such as sleep apnea and restless leg syndrome or psychological causes such as depression or anxiety.

One of the biggest problems people face is handling stress. I have dealt with many patients throughout my medical practice who have come to me with severe stress reactions to daily challenges. The perception of something as a life stress is often more dependent on how the individual *perceives* stress than on the event itself. When faced with life-and-death situations, such as health crises, some people feel challenged by the situation while others may be paralyzed with fear.

Severe stress reactions can cause real physical illness, such as heart attacks, strokes, and ulcers. Many feel that dealing with life comes down to *attitude*. Attitude is how you perceive, react to, and deal with life.

Your doctor may inquire how stressful you perceive your life to be. You may need to modify your coping mechanisms to preserve your health. I had a recent epiphany, which is simply being able to *overlook things that are of no major consequence.*

Furthermore, I'm trying to be actually *be happy with things I don't agree with and/or cannot change!* There are several techniques that one can try to accomplish this.

There are situations in life that are truly terrible and are difficult to deal with for anyone. A lovely hospital worker came home one evening to find her house had burned down and her daughters, ages thirteen and fifteen, had perished. I witnessed her dark-brown hair turn gray within two weeks. After many months and interventions with this unfortunate woman, I helped her move out of this anguished mental state. This, along with the other interventions, helped her to a degree.

There are important lessons to be learned from this. There are worse situations than yours or mine, and stress can affect the body in many ways never thought about.

You can go to any large bookstore and find a book you think may help your individual situation. Self-awareness, psychological consulting, biofeedback, hypnosis, yoga, and relaxation techniques may be utilized. Many feel it all comes down to what we are talking about, and that is *attitude.* Attitude is how you perceive, react to, and deal with life. *Overlooking and trying to be happy with stressors and things you cannot change* will help you in many ways!

Holistic physicians encourage patients to evoke the healing power of love, hope, enthusiasm, and humor to release the toxic consequences of hostility, shame, greed, depression, and prolonged fear, anger, and grief. Several patients—and I personally—have experienced the positive power of laughter.

It can instantaneously change your perspective, mood, and reactions to a situation in a positive way.

I think laughter may release, as does exercise, natural opioids and various hormones that make you feel good and are health promoting. The "runner's high" is thought to be caused by the body's natural release of opioids, and I believe hormones (testosterone and growth hormone, both of which are medically proven to elevate with exercise) are also released.

An important part of your visit with your alternative-medicine clinician should include a discussion of your diet. Your diet should be rich in natural, raw, high-density foods such as leafy green vegetables, fruits, and whole grains, and if you eat animal products, free-range or organic-fed meats and poultry are the best to consume. The opposite of high-density foods include empty calorie foods such as soda, candy, ice cream, and highly sweetened foods (e.g., high concentrations of sugar, or *any amount* of high fructose corn syrup). Regarding these last two "foods": *if it's man-made, don't eat it!*

You should eat only what your body needs. You can adjust your intake to your needs. For instance, if you are jogging longer distances than usual, you will need to consume more carbohydrates. If you are not very active, you should consume fewer carbohydrates. Many diabetics who take insulin administer their dose on a "sliding" scale—that is, they can manipulate their dose to match their diet and activity level. For example, if you are weightlifting more than usual, you may need to increase your protein intake. Your diet can be a major determinant to your health. Obesity and malnutrition are closely linked to the development of diabetes, heart disease, bone disease, and other ailments.

This author believes a vegetarian diet tends to be healthier; however, this is difficult to isolate as a sole reason for better health. Vegetarians tend to exercise more, and often do not smoke or consume a lot of alcohol. These healthy lifestyle habits could be reasons for better health of the vegetarian. For excellent information on the benefits of vegetarianism, visit www.vegetarian-nutrition.com.

The December 19, 2011, *New York Times* article featured the benefits of a healthy lifestyle as it tied into longevity. The focus was on town of Loma Linda, California. This small city has a large Seventh-Day Adventist community who are primarily vegetarians. This community has one of the highest longevity rates in the world according to some statistics, and healthy lifestyle habits are also attributed as contributing factors. This article features heart surgeon Dr. Ellsworth Wareham, who is ninety-seven years old and stopped working only two years ago! He has been a vegan for the past thirty or forty years. This town dissuades the consumption of meat, smoking, and drinking alcohol.

The August 31, 2009, *Time* magazine article "The Real Cost of Cheap Food" describes the terrible condition farms are kept in and how convenience foods are dreadfully unhealthy. I believe there is a huge difference between eating unhealthy animals as opposed to free-range and organically or grass-fed animals, and it can have a great impact on one's health.

It is vital to *drink eight or more glasses of distilled water per day.* It should be noted that not all water is equal. You could have your tap water tested for contaminants such as heavy metals, pesticides, insecticides, benzene, bacteria, etc. There are many effective water filters available for the entire house and/or drinking water, preferably a reverse-osmosis system.

Bottled water should not be an option. Some feel that if the bottle is exposed to heat or cold, the plastic breaks down and causes chemicals to leach out. Environmentalists feel plastic bottles add to the waste problem.

Water intake should also be adjusted to suit your activity level and the environmental conditions. On average, one should drink eight to ten glasses of water a day. Beverages containing caffeine and/or alcohol are not a desirable substitute for water because they can cause excessive urination, resulting in water depletion. I recommend visiting www.watercure.com for more information.

Your doctor may question you about the type of exercise you do. Both anaerobic (resistance/strength building) and aerobic (jogging, biking) should be utilized at every age. Regular exercise has been scientifically proven to decrease heart disease, cancer, dementia, obesity, inflammatory molecules, osteoporosis, and physical disabilities. In addition, exercise produces increased energy and an overall improved sense of well-being.

An exercise program should also exercise the brain. Studies provide hope that certain areas of the brain can regenerate, notably the areas responsible for Alzheimer's disease. See "Exercise-Induced Neuronal Plasticity in Central Autonomic

Networks: Role in Cardiovascular Control" by Lisete C. Michelini and Javier E. Stem, published in *Exp Physiol.* 94, no. 9 (Sept. 2009): 947–60 and in the *Proceedings of the National Academy of Sciences*, May 2004.

It is fascinating to postulate that mental and physical exercise could aid in brain regeneration. My mother-in-law reads constantly and does crossword puzzles to keep her brain sharp, and she is dangerously quick-witted!

You should make exercise an enjoyable activity. It shouldn't be, as one patient called it, "dedicated torture"! Because several of my patients find it difficult to exercise, I call it "the hardest vitamin pill to swallow." Make it enjoyable through music, a good atmosphere, by working out with friends and/or a trainer, and utilizing the different types of exercise that agree with you.

Make exercise interesting and enjoyable at all times!

No discussion about a healthy lifestyle would be complete without mentioning smoking cessation. Years ago, before we knew the health consequences of smoking, it seemed as if everybody smoked. If you watch any movie from the 1930s to the 1970s, it seems like everybody smoked. Subsequently, the true health hazards of smoking were revealed. We now know of the direct toxic effects of smoking and the correlation between smoking and diseases of the heart, blood vessels, and lungs, and the incidence of certain cancers.

It is understandable how people who have been smoking for many years can have a difficult time stopping, as smoking is an addiction. Some people incorrectly believe that the damage has been done and stopping smoking will not improve their health. Smoking cessation can and does halt the progression of vascular disease and can cause disease regression.

I am still baffled by the younger generation—today's teenagers. Despite the fact that they are exposed to a multitude of media sources (most of which many of us have never even heard of), they squander the opportunity to educate themselves in regard to the harmful side effects of smoking, and continue to do so. In fact, the amount of teenagers who smoke is still on the rise. I am appalled when I pick up my daughter from her high school and see the cloud of smoke emanating from the area right outside the school. Perhaps teenagers feel some false sense of immortality, or an overly optimistic view of their health.

Unfortunately, for the young, getting old is just distant rumor, being diseased is just a myth, and planning for either is not considered.

Finally, you and your physician are partners in your health care. Your relationship with your doctor is key. There should be trust in your physician and a relationship that is comfortable enough for you to ask questions about your health and treatment. In my practice, I give my patients a pad to take notes so they remember what we discussed, and often they get homework so they can read and understand the plan that has been personalized for them. There are now so many articles on health care and antiaging strategies available. I encourage you to read *Life Extension* magazine for many different medical points of view (http://www.lef.org/magazine/).

Based on the patient's response to treatment, the plan will either remain the same or will be modified. As everyone is genetically and physiologically different, each individual will have his or her own response to a given treatment plan. The physician and the patient must both be open-minded and realize that sometimes things don't work optimally the first time around. A good example of this is blood pressure medicine. Different drugs work well on different people. I constantly hear frustration from patients who have poorly controlled blood pressure and require multiple trials with different drugs before they find their blood pressure under control.

A friend recently contacted her new doctor's office so her prescriptions could be renewed. The patient had expected to receive written prescriptions for the same medications that she had been taking, some of them for years. The physician's office called the prescriptions in to the pharmacy to make things easier for the patient. When she picked up her prescriptions, she was both surprised and dismayed to find out that most of the medications had been changed to similar drugs without informing her.

In addition, she had a long history of medication reactions and unpleasant side effects that made her unable to tolerate several of these drugs. She was confused and uncertain about what to do. Was this the fault of the patient or the physician? I say both.

While the physician should have consulted with the patient to determine whether she had had prior negative reactions to these medications, the patient should have made it clear during her medical evaluation that she had a history of multiple drug reactions and which drugs she could not tolerate. The doctor-patient relationship must be an open partnership. I have found it true that two heads are definitely better than one! Health care is dynamic, not static, so the treatment plan must constantly be reevaluated.

In summary, the following can serve as helpful tips to help maximize your healthy lifestyle and ultimately your overall health:

❖ Eat a healthy, balanced diet consisting only of what your body needs.

    ➢ What is a good diet?
- high density foods (low calorie, high vitamin, protein, mineral foods)
- raw, organic grains, vegetables, and fruits
- primarily vegetarian: protein from nuts, seeds, and beans; if desired, include fish, poultry, and low-fat or nonfat dairy; limit amounts of lean red meat (if consumed); organic, free range produce is preferred.
- drinking at least 8-10 glasses of pure water per day
- eating only what you need; body weight equals what you eat minus what you expend.

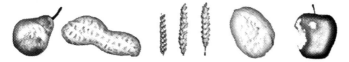

❖ Maintain a positive attitude.

❖ Exercise regularly.

❖ Sleep well and adequately.

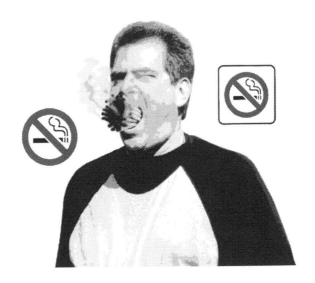

❖ Do not smoke.

❖ Do not drink alcohol to excess (if any).

❖ Maintain healthy interpersonal relationships.

❖ Control the stress in your life.

❖ Schedule regular medical checkups.

❖ Relax and have fun.

WebMD.com offers numerous articles on the benefits of the Mediterranean Diet. Start with "Popular Diets of the World: The Mediterranean Diet" (http://www.webmd.com/diet/features/the-Mediterranean-diet), "Mediterranean Diet Plus

Exercise Cuts Alzheimer's Risk" (http://www.webmd.com/alzheimers/news/20090811/mediterranean-diet-plus-exercise-cuts-alzheimers-risk), and "Benefits of the Mediterranean Diet: A delicious Mediterranean eating plan can help protect against heart disease, diabetes, cancer—even help with weight loss" (http://www.webmd.com/diet/features/benefits-mediterranean-diet). This website offers many well-referenced articles on several topics mentioned or discussed in this book. I highly recommend it for a source of knowledge and medical references.

> *If we could give every individual the right amount of*
> *nourishment and exercise, not too little and not too much,*
> *we would have found the safest way to health.*
> —Hippocrates

> *When it comes to eating right and exercising, there is no*
> *"I'll start tomorrow." Tomorrow is disease.*
> —Terri Guillemets

CHAPTER 5

CARDIOVASCULAR DISEASE

According to the Centers for Disease Control and Prevention (CDC), heart disease is the leading cause of morbidity (disease) and mortality (death) in the United States (http://www.cdc.gov/heartdisease/statistics.htm).

Atherosclerosis, the progressive narrowing in medium- and large-sized arteries from deposits of lipids and calcium, is increasing in prevalence in developing countries. In recent years, age-related mortality attributable to atherosclerosis has been decreasing; however, cerebral vascular atherosclerosis (affecting the brain) and heart disease still cause greater than 650,000 annual deaths in the United States (almost six times more than accidents and is more common than cancer). The incidence of atherosclerosis will continue to increase, and it is predicted that by the year 2020, atherosclerosis will be the leading cause of death worldwide (http://www.cdc.gov/heartdisease/statistics.htm).

Until recently, arteries were considered to be simply tubes that carried the blood. It was not recognized that they are living, dynamic tissue that go through changes over time. Heart and peripheral vascular disease are developmental processes. They do not occur overnight or in mysterious ways. The buildup of cholesterol (and other substances, such as clotting factors, platelets, calcium forms, inflammatory cells, connective tissue, and smooth muscle from the arterial wall itself) eventually form what has been called "hardening of the arteries," plaque, and atherosclerosis. The buildup of this plaque causes a narrowing within the artery.

This results in decreased blood and oxygen to the supplied area such as the heart, brain, and other vital organs. It is like stepping on a garden hose, decreasing the flow of water to the sprinkler. Eventually the reduced flow from the blockage causes tissue to lose its blood supply and may cause cell death in the area supplied by the artery unless acute medical intervention takes place to block this process.

How does the body know, for example, that there is an acute process going on in the heart? One of the body's defenses is pain. The sensation of pain lets the brain know that there is something wrong. The patient may experience chest pain, nausea, sweating, and shortness of breath. This is called angina. It is often dismissed by the patient as "indigestion." It can initially occur during exercise. Narrowing of the arteries can be looked at in terms of "supply and demand."

When you exercise, you put more demand on your arteries and your heart, which in some people may have an insufficient blood supply. In rare cases, this can acutely lead to a heart attack, stroke. In the chronic setting, this can cause peripheral vascular disease (e.g., skin infections, ulcer, or gangrene).

Since this process is developmental, it is an opportunity for us to be proactive and prevent this deadly process. This is why it is recommended that you should always consult with your primary care physician (PCP) before beginning any exercise regimen. Let your doctor give you a clean bill of health before you begin.

There are several risk factors for the development of atherosclerosis. They include dyslipidemia (e.g., lipid fat/cholesterol abnormalities); diabetes; cigarette smoking; family history; hypertension; sedentary lifestyle; obesity; excessive stress; oxidative stressors (e.g., free radicals such as superoxide and hydroxyl, which form molecular bonds with cholesterol and other fats, causing them to form a coating [plaque] within the artery, resulting in decreased blood flow and oxygen. Free radicals attack other cellular components, causing damage. They are one of the known causes of aging).

Inflammation (e.g., elevated C-reactive protein [CRP] and homocysteine); infection (e.g., dental infections, sinusitis, prostatitis, fungal infections); elevated clotting factors; uric acid; heavy metals (e.g., aluminum, mercury, and lead); and advanced age have been connected to heart disease.

Mainstream medicine has made numerous advances in prevention, diagnosis, and treatment of cardiovascular disease. Recent advances include educating patients regarding diet, exercise, and other lifestyle issues. It is also recommended that patients maintain tight control over their diabetes, hypertension, and cholesterol profiles and give up detrimental habits such as smoking and excessively drinking alcohol.

However, due to time restraints, your primary care physician (PCP) and/or cardiologist are typically unable to devote ample time to counsel patients in a detailed fashion as to why they might be overweight, smoking, and/or not exercising. Some medical doctors realize they have limited time and refer their patients to appropriate clinicians to deal with these issues in a more complete fashion.

The alternative integrative/complementary practitioner, typically, has more time to devote to such issues. Be that as it may, indeed, standard medical care now recognizes it is involved with the importance of lifestyle changes, as it has realized their importance in impacting heart health and other health issues.

Modern medicine uses several important diagnostic tools regarding heart disease. This includes the "usual and customary" physical exam; a complete cholesterol profile; an EKG; stress testing (whether a standard stress test or with the addition of a "nuclear agent," such as technetium 99) to look for signs of significant blockages in the coronary arteries; an echocardiogram to evaluate the function and structure of the heart and its valves; and, when indicated, an angiogram to delineate "exact coronary artery anatomy" (blood vessels supplying the heart with blood and oxygen).

Angiography (radiologic method of visualizing arteries) regarding the heart is called cardiac catheterization. This is traditionally done by injecting a radio-opaque contrast agent into blood vessels, and it is the most sensitive tool used in diagnosing coronary artery disease.

Another cardiac diagnostic tool is the Holter monitor (or just "Holter"), which is a portable device the patient wears that continuously monitors various electrical activity of the heart. This can diagnose cardiac arrhythmias (when the heart is not beating normally). Other tools utilized are CT scans, echocardiograms, or MRIs of the heart.

Once disease of a coronary artery is diagnosed, a stent (an artificial "tube") can be placed within the artery to increase blood flow and prevent a heart attack. In the event of severe multivessel disease or severe disease of the heart valves, surgery may be a viable option.

But what can we do medically to prevent heart disease before it happens? We have already briefly discussed modification or reduction of risk factors such as obesity and smoking. Cholesterol should be monitored, starting with a complete lipid profile, which should include total cholesterol, LDL (low density lipoprotein, or "bad" cholesterol), triglycerides, HDL (high density lipoprotein, or "good" cholesterol), and the LDL: HDL ratio. Higher levels of HDL are protective against atherosclerotic heart disease. Elevated total cholesterol or LDL can cause heart disease.

There are also subsets of the HDL and LDL molecules, which can be measured (using what is called a VAP test) and aid in preventing and/or treating vascular disease. What might appear to be a high and healthy HDL may actually not be so! The large, buoyant, protective type of HDL may actually be low, and the small, dense, less protective HDL particle can be elevated! Therefore, what appeared to be a normal or an elevated total HDL (add both the small dense and the large buoyant HDL) is in essence not protective and can put the patient at risk for heart disease. When just a total HDL is obtained, this can be missed.

Cholesterol medicines and alternative therapies are aimed toward reducing total cholesterol and LDL and to elevate HDL levels. There is no longer one number that should be considered everyone's LDL or HDL cholesterol goal. Someone who has a history of heart disease or many risk factors for heart disease needs to be kept under tighter control than someone who is young and free of disease and risk factors.

Some patients are able to drastically change their lifestyles and make a profound positive effect on their cholesterol profiles, so much so that they do not require medications. Unfortunately, some patients are adherent to a low-cholesterol diet but still require medication. There are several specific diet plans and natural therapies available for correcting cholesterol profiles. Several supplements and foods such as red yeast rice, niacin, lecithin, omega-3, garlic, leafy green vegetables, and oatmeal can be beneficial.

On the negative side, natural therapies typically require taking several doses and/or different products throughout the day. Failure to respond to natural products can be due to self-medicating. Correct dosing and combining of natural products and/or medications can make the difference between treatment failure and success. Some patients cannot tolerate this and would rather take the pharmaceutical once a day that "does the trick." Conventional treatment relies heavily on the use of statin medicines to treat cholesterol.

The efficacy of statin medications in treating high cholesterol and in stabilizing plaques in arteries has been established in many studies. They have been proven to decrease cholesterol and stabilize plaque. Their use can be limited by unpleasant side effects, including muscle and liver disorders. There is also some concern that statin drugs may inhibit the neuroprotective effects of the substance Coenzyme Q (CoQ10), resulting in worsening dementia; however, more studies are needed in this area.

Statin drugs and red yeast rice can lower CoQ10 levels in the body. This author recommends taking CoQ10 when on either red yeast rice or statin drugs. I obtain CoQ10 blood levels on my patients taking either statin drugs or red yeast rice. Blood testing guides the dosing of CoQ10 in a scientific fashion, as with thyroid hormone replacement.

One recent article, "Simvastatin versus Therapeutic Lifestyle Changes and Supplements: Randomized Primary Prevention Trial," published in *Mayo Clinic Proceedings* in July 2008, found that lifestyle changes, combined with ingestion of the supplements red yeast rice and fish oil reduced LDL cholesterol in similar proportion to simvastatin (Zocor), one of the statin medications routinely used to lower cholesterol.

And the January 15, 2010, article "Tolerability of Red Yeast Rice (2,400 mg Twice Daily) versus Pravastatin (20 mg Twice Daily) in Patients with Previous Statin Intolerance," published in *The American Journal of Cardiology*, drew the conclusion that "red yeast rice was tolerated as well as pravastatin and achieved a comparable reduction of low-density lipoprotein cholesterol in a population previously intolerant to statins." Actually, red yeast rice fared slightly better in lowering low-density lipoprotein (LDL) than the statin drug. LDL decreased 30 percent for the red yeast group and 27 percent for the statin group.

When evaluating risk factors for heart disease, a blood panel (a full "blood exam," or workup) looking for inflammatory markers should be performed. It has been documented that elevated levels of C-reactive protein, and in some studies elevated homocysteine, can cause heart disease.

In fact C-reactive protein, when elevated, can accelerate the formation of atherosclerosis and cause a rupture of the plaque. Metal ions such as copper and possibly other heavy metals (including aluminum, lead, and mercury) can act as inflammatory agents, causing atherosclerosis. Natural methods to "chelate"—remove potentially toxic metals—are discussed later in the book.

When a piece of atherosclerotic plaque flakes off (ruptures), it travels down a blood vessel until it cannot continue due to the narrow width of the blood vessel. It will block the blood flow at this point, therefore affecting whatever tissue is beyond it, which will die as the result of a heart attack or stroke.

It is my opinion that C-reactive protein and homocysteine should be included in baseline blood tests. If a level is elevated, it should be treated and then retested after treatment has been initiated. Present medical recommendation is to obtain these tests when indicated (dependent upon a patient's age and risk factors), but this is considered a special request. I have found several patients with significantly elevated levels. They didn't fit into the "risk group," so the tests weren't performed. Therefore, I would recommend that you discuss the utilization of these tests with your physician.

Homocysteine can be lowered by taking B12, folate, and trimethylglycine, and by diet modifications (decreasing red meat intake). The cause of elevated C-reactive protein (CRP) should be treated whenever possible. Chronic infection such as sinusitis, prostatitis, urinary tract, and dental infections should be looked into, since they can elevate CRP. Vitamin C, fish oil, and aspirin have been approved by traditional medicine to lower CRP. If these are ineffective, pycnogenol (a natural anti-inflammatory and antioxidant) should be tried.

Another important test is lipoprotein (a) (Lp (a)), which doesn't respond to statin-type drugs. Niacin (vitamin B3) is approved for the elevated Lp (a). Other blood tests such as fibrinogen, uric acid, anticardiolipin antibodies, and antithrombin III could be helpful in identifying an at-risk-for-cardiovascular-disease patient. If you don't have medical insurance and would like to have a detailed blood test, Life Extension (www.lef.org) offers major discounts (see the references/resources section at the end of this book for more information).

There are several other natural substances that should be considered regarding the prevention and treatment of heart disease. It is now medically accepted to use fish oils. There are many articles indicating that fish oils can decrease heart disease, stroke, dementia, and other health conditions. To date, there is only one FDA-approved pharmaceutical fish oil, called Lovaza. I have used this preparation with success in many regards. Niacin is also called vitamin B3. It has been used for many years, pioneered by alternative medicine, and later by mainstream medicine. It can be used to treat low HDL, and high triglycerides, total cholesterol, and LDL levels.

It is medically accepted that using omega-3 fish oil supplements reduces triglycerides and elevates the "good" cholesterol HDL. Unfortunately, some over-the-counter fish oils may contain heavy metals such as mercury. Clearly, mercury-free preparations should be utilized. This is why I use the pharmaceutical grade whenever possible. These tend to be purer in form.

Several medications can prevent the formation of clots and atherosclerosis. Such medicines, to use the lay term, are classified as blood thinners. These include aspirin, heparin, warfarin, clopidogrel, lovenox, tissue plasminogen activator, and others. These medicines have helped thousands upon thousands either in an acute setting (heart attack, stroke, blood clot) or in preventing heart attacks, strokes, and peripheral vascular disease.

Natural therapeutics in health and disease can have numerous benefits. A low-fat diet has been shown to offer many health benefits. The article, "Can Lifestyle Changes Reverse Coronary Heart Disease? The Lifestyle Heart Trial," conducted by Dr. Dean Ornish and published by *The Lancet*, promotes utilizing a very low-fat, whole food, vegetarian diet high in complex carbohydrates and low in simple sugars along with cessation of smoking, increased exercise (walking), and stress management techniques. It has demonstrated a 91 percent reduction in frequency of angina and the regression of coronary atherosclerosis after only one year, with even more regression after five years.

Antioxidants have also been recommended since oxidation of cholesterol can accelerate the atherosclerotic process. However, an article indicated that four hundred units of vitamin E (D-alpha tocopherol) actually had negative effects. "Meta-Analysis: High-Dosage Vitamin E Supplementation May Increase All-Cause Mortality," published in the *Annals of Internal Medicine*, caused several debates.

It was felt by alternative practitioners that the vitamin E that was utilized was not a natural and complete form of vitamin E. Vitamin E has several "family members" that were omitted. There is also a sister molecule called tocotrenole, which was not utilized within the vitamin E study. When using only the D-alpha tocopherol and not the other types (such as gamma, delta, zeta, etc.), the effect to the body would not be favorable.

Unfortunately, only a few vitamin companies have taken this information into account in their formation of appropriate vitamin E products. Many well-written and well-referenced articles have been published on this subject and other interesting health-related issues by the Life Extension Foundation in their monthly journal (see the references section at the end of this book).

There are other studies showing the benefits of antioxidants having a positive effect on atherosclerosis and other health issues. A standard medical journal called *Circulation* recommended in 2003 the use of antioxidants prior to exercise since potentially damaging free radicals are created when exercising.

There is also a well-known study called the Nurse's Health Study, founded in 1976, which studied the health of 238,000 dedicated nurse-participants. The study found that individuals with the highest dietary intake of vitamin E had about a 40 percent reduction in cardiovascular disease risk.

Another point to consider is that the dietary form of vitamin E is consumed in its whole food, natural form. There is no substitute for whole foods. There are substances occurring in nature that have proven beneficial, although we do not fully understand their usefulness yet. This is an important concept that encourages one to live a healthy lifestyle and include raw, natural foods on a daily basis.

In 1996, after conducting its study "Randomized Controlled Trial of Vitamin E in Patients with Coronary Disease: Cambridge Heart Antioxidant Study (CHAOS)," the Cambridge Heart Antioxidant Study published its findings in *The Lancet.* It showed the health benefits of antioxidants and discovered that vitamin E reduced the risk of nonfatal myocardial infarction in patients suffering from established coronary artery disease.

Other studies showing that antioxidants were not effective regarding the prevention of coronary artery disease (*New England Journal of Medicine* 330 (1994): 1029; *New England Journal of Medicine* 337 (1997): 365) should be considered, since nothing is absolute. Even antioxidants and supplements can be harmful or even toxic when not properly utilized. Excessive use of antioxidants can actually cause a pro-oxidant state and cause harm! *Too much can be as bad as too little!* For example, while it is well known that populations that are primarily vegetarian do not smoke, are not obese, have active lifestyles, and often have less cardiovascular diseases (the Christian Scientists and Seventh-Day Adventists are good examples of this), by isolating various vitamins, one could be leaving out important substances and combinations, causing more harm than good.

In fact, beta-carotene should not be utilized in excess with patients who smoke since it can actually increase the incidence of lung cancer. Therefore, adding isolated vitamins isn't a substitute for a healthy lifestyle and may actually be harmful. Again, I would caution against self-medicating. One should go to a practitioner who is familiar with the studies regarding vitamins so that appropriate combinations can be utilized in a scientific fashion for a positive, not negative, effect.

Coenzyme Q (CoQ) 10, or ubiquinone, is an important molecule in the treatment of heart disease. CoQ10 is involved in energy production (it is required in the cells' mitochondria for oxidative phosphorylation and the production of ATP, which is a multifunctional nucleotide used in cells as a coenzyme). This is extremely important since the heart muscle (myocardium) is composed of high-energy tissue.

The heart does not rest unless it has stopped, which of course is not a desirable event! CoQ is also an important antioxidant and works in a synergistic or additive fashion with vitamin E to reduce the oxidation of LDL cholesterol. The oxidation of LDL is thought to be a major cause in the development of atherosclerosis.

Another important aspect of CoQ is the fact that statin drugs inhibit an enzyme that makes cholesterol but also inhibits CoQ10. It is, therefore, recommended by alternative practitioners and some mainstream medical physicians to give CoQ10 supplements to patients taking statin drugs. CoQ10 lab results from two large companies (Lab Cor and Quest Labs) will state that CoQ10 levels greater than 2.5 have been found to be cardio-protective.

Hypertension (high blood pressure) is now being treated in a more aggressive and proactive fashion by mainstream medicine. Studies reveal which medicines have an effect on mortality and morbidity and not just report their ability to lower blood pressure. Years ago, limited medications meant some patients' high blood pressure would be difficult to manage.

There are many different hypertension medications available. It is rare that a patient cannot have adequate blood pressure control, unless there are structural reasons for the high blood pressure, such as diseases affecting the arteries to the kidneys (renal artery stenosis).

Medical diseases that cause high blood pressure are thoroughly investigated when *uncontrolled* blood pressure occurs in young people or in people who are compliant regarding combination therapy involving multiple drugs. If a patient has borderline hypertension (e.g., 140/86), standard medical care, as would the alternative practitioner most likely, would recommend a trial of lifestyle change.

This should include all parameters of a healthy lifestyle. One should lose appropriate weight (primarily fat weight). A low-sodium diet and increasing water intake (see www. watercure.com) should be recommended. Daily cardiovascular exercise, which increases the heart rate for at least twenty minutes, is advised and should be prescribed and overseen by a practitioner familiar with exercise physiology (e.g., cardiologist or sports medicine specialist). Please note that patients should also be cautious when initiating an exercise program, as too much too soon can cause injury and may exacerbate preexisting medical conditions.

Electrolytes such as magnesium and potassium are known to help lower blood pressure. If one has blood tests that reveal that their magnesium and potassium levels are low or within the lower limits of normal, one should try to elevate them into the mid, if not high, normal limits. Low or elevated levels can also cause other problems such as muscle weakness or abnormal heart rhythms.

Typically in mainstream medicine, when someone is diagnosed with high blood pressure, he or she is started on a diuretic (water pill). These are notorious for decreasing blood levels of potassium and magnesium. Therefore, your doctor will typically order blood tests shortly after starting you on this type of medicine.

One should also avoid products such as ephedra and yohimbine supplements, since these herbal products can elevate blood pressure. More conventional medicines, such as decongestants (allergy and other medicines if a decongestant was added) and anti-inflammatory medicines (such as ibuprofen), either prescribed or over-the-counter can also elevate blood pressure. It is important to speak to your doctor before starting any medicines and herbals.

Conventional medicine treatment of the heart and blood vessels has been well established. Alternative therapeutics, when applied in scientific and logical fashion, offer several benefits. They may enable a patient to avoid the use of conventional medicines, reduce the amount of his current medicines, help buffer the side effects of the medicine, and/or potentiate the medications in a positive fashion. Additionally, they may decrease the actual disease process and its concurrent symptoms.

As I will stress many times in this book, using several different disease states as examples, it is my opinion that the successful combination of conventional and alternative approaches provides an additive benefit in treating disease and in the overall well being of the individual. However, you should be guided by a physician who understands and practices integrative medicine.

CHAPTER 6
CANCER

One-third of the population in the United States will eventually develop cancer. Clearly it is a monumental health and economic problem. The percentage of people dying from cancer is increasing, as the population ages and death from cardiovascular disease declines.

The general definition of cancer is that it originates from genetic changes in a single cell that proliferates to form a clone of malignant cells; cancer cell growth is not properly regulated by the normal biochemical and physical influences in the environment; cancer cells have the capacity to spread away from their site of origin and spread throughout the body. "Cancer" is a general term that describes the process, but each type of cancer behaves in a different way, depending on the location and the specific molecular products of the cancer.

Each type of cancer follows a relatively distinct natural course. Some cancers spread, for example, to the lungs, others to bone and brain. Some cancers are slow growing and others are aggressive. In order to develop a treatment plan, it is important to know the type of cancer and the natural history of the cancer, including its typical rate of growth. Some cancers are amenable to one modality approach, while others must be treated aggressively with a multimodality approach (*you cannot hold back an ocean with one spoon*).

Basal cell and squamous carcinoma of the skin, and some early stage 1 and 2 cancers, can be treated with rapid surgical excision, as this approach results in a high cure rate. Most advanced stage 4 (where the cancer has spread to multiple areas of the body) cancers require multimodality treatment.

Before discussing specific treatments for cancer, it is important to consider those factors that may be responsible for causing cancer, be they internal or environmental. First, genetic factors play an important role. Clearly some families have a predisposition toward certain types of cancers. The importance of knowing genetic predisposition for a cancer is that screening for disease in asymptomatic persons must be more aggressive. Breast cancer is a good example.

It is known that certain families have a high incidence of breast cancer. Some women possess a gene known as BRCA, which is highly linked to breast (and ovarian) cancer. The presence of this gene in someone with the right family history and an at-risk ethnic background (Ashkenazi Jewish ancestry) would prompt earlier and more aggressive surveillance.

Exposure to a wide variety of environmental toxins can cause cancer. For example, exposure to radiation, benzene, heavy metals, asbestosis, and high electrical voltage exposure has been linked to the development of cancer. The most sensitive tissues are the bone marrow, breast, and thyroid. Patients who have received radiation for other cancers may develop leukemia (a disease of the blood and bone marrow) several years later, as may those individuals treated with certain cancer chemotherapies known as alkylating agents.

Sun exposure is the primary risk factor in skin cancer, most notably in fair-skinned individuals. Obviously, avoidance of excessive amounts of direct sun and the use of protective clothing and sunscreen will lessen the incidence.

There are multiple other exposures that are linked to cancer, such as asbestos (exposure resulting in mesothelioma), arsenic, benzene, and polycyclic hydrocarbons. While tobacco smoking is clearly linked to lung cancer, it is also associated with increased incidence of cancers of the oral cavity, esophagus, kidney, bladder, and pancreas.

There is also the phenomenon of "passive smoking." Smoking in the presence of your family and loved ones puts them at risk for the toxic effects of inhaled smoke. I will never forget seeing a woman pushing a baby in a stroller with her lit cigarette dangling at the level of the baby's face. This is hardly a healthy outing for the baby's lungs. There are many choices available now for people to help them stop smoking. You should review your options with your doctor.

There have also been studies on the role of diet and nutrition and their impact on cancer. Diets that are low in fat, include fruits and whole cereal fiber, avoid consumption of salt-cured and smoked food, and use alcohol in moderation are not only nutritionally sound but may decrease the incidence of various types of cancers.

There are many *unidentified or unclassified causes and/or risk factors that attribute to the development of cancer and other diseases.*

CONVENTIONAL CANCER TREATMENT

As previously discussed, there is no magic cure for most cancers. Treatment in general depends on the cancer's type, location, and its natural history (e.g., how aggressively the cancer will spread and invade other body organs). Cancer may be categorized as a "stage," which usually defines the outermost border, and size. Cancer can be confined to one location (stage I–II), spread to adjacent tissues (stage III), or widely spread to other areas of the body (stage IV).

The first modality used to treat cancer, dating back to the nineteenth century, was surgery. Frequently, a surgical piece of tissue or a biopsy is needed to determine the type of cancer the patient has. Surgical procedures are done to determine the stage, cell type, other pathological information, and to remove the cancer. Some cancers may be surgically removed as a definitive treatment, or as part of a treatment plan that combines with other modalities such as chemotherapy and/or radiation.

Radiation therapy, like surgery, treats the cancer locally. The goal is to destroy cancerous tissue with minimal damage to the surrounding normal tissue. Sometimes radiation may be delivered by insertion of radioactive materials into the body. DNA in the cancer cell is the target for radiation-induced cell death.

Ionizing radiation generates free radicals and reactive oxygen intermediates that cause damage to local cell components including DNA. This is why antioxidants such as vitamins C and E, selenium, glutathione, carcinoids, and others should be timed appropriately when using radiation and some chemotherapeutic agents as they can *interfere* with their efficacy.

Rapidly growing cancer cells and normal cells (skin, bone marrow) are the most susceptible to radiation and chemotherapy. Radiation therapy may be curative as a sole treatment in certain types of cancers, or it may be used as part of a treatment regimen on others. It may also be used as palliative therapy to relieve pain in certain types of bone cancers, or to relieve swelling in cancers of the brain and nervous system.

Sometimes chemotherapy and/or radiation are given prior to surgery. This is called neo-adjuvant therapy. This is done to possibly reduce the size of the cancer; therefore, the surgical procedure is a lesser one. This presurgical approach may also reduce cancer cells from leaching out of the surgical site and spreading to other areas of the body.

Finally, systemic chemotherapy is the primary treatment for widespread disease, even if the primary site of the cancer is not known. Certain cancers may be cured by chemotherapy; in others, there may be some beneficial activity when used in combination with surgery and radiation.

Chemotherapeutic regimens work in different ways. Most are toxic to actively dividing cells; some are toxic to cells at rest that have not actively multiplied. A complete discussion of the various types of chemotherapy and the cancers they treat should be discussed on an individual basis by the patient and his or her doctor.

Almost all of the chemotherapeutic agents display a "dose-response" effect, which means that these agents become more toxic to both normal and cancer cells with higher dosages. This eventually leads to a plateau where higher doses are not more beneficial in treatment but clearly create more untoward side effects.

Chemotherapy is typically given in cycles. The number of cycles is determined by the protocol itself, the patient's response, and the side effects experienced by the patient. Sometimes chemotherapy can cause nausea, vomiting, weakness, anemia, and susceptibility to infection.

As we are treating an individual and not a disease, the patient and the physician must communicate with each other and weigh the benefits of treatment and the risks of unpleasant side effects. There are several things available in both traditional and alternative medicine that can buffer the side effects of treatment.

When there is a suspicion of a cancer or a biopsy-proven diagnosis, time is generally crucial in developing a treatment plan to prevent the spread of the cancer. Typically, the patient is referred to an oncologist for further management. The oncologist will determine, if possible, the type of cancer, the degree of spread, and the natural history of the cancer. They will then plan a course of action utilizing some combination of the aforementioned treatment modalities.

Practitioners, who have knowledge of alternative therapies, may utilize, when appropriate additional treatment modalities, some of which will be described later. Alternative therapies may include life style changes, detoxification, immune system enhancement, specific oral and intravenous nutritional therapies, controlled amino acid therapy (caat), hydrogen peroxide, B17, hyperthermia, hormonal manipulation, ozone, chemotherapy sensitivity analysis, Insulin Potentiation Therapy (IPT), and many others.

Conventional cancer treatments bring with them extensive scientific testing and documentation of efficacy. Some treatments may prove successful in only a small population size. If a drug is found to be successful, for example, 5 percent of the time, how can we be sure this is from the chemotherapeutic agent and is not just a placebo effect or something that occurs by chance? Using large study populations in conventional medical trials can help eliminate these factors.

Scientific testing for alternative cancer therapies is not always available. There are several reasons for this, typically arising from financial constraints. As alternative treatments are generally inexpensive and cannot be patented, drug companies have no incentive to pursue these treatments. Additional government and funding institutions do not tend to allocate money to alternative research. It is also possible with any type of cancer for spontaneous remission with little treatment to attribute this to, whether with conventional or alternative methods.

Alternative cancer treatments are generally prescribed in addition to conventional cancer treatments and not in lieu of them. It is important to realize that combining these treatments *should only be administered by practitioners who are well versed in both methods of care!* Negative side effects, including treatment failure, can result from improper combinations.

Used correctly, alternative therapies can potentiate conventional cancer treatments and increase their success rate. The general well-being and health of the individual can also be improved by such means as nutritional support, hormonal manipulation, and immune system enhancement when indicated.

As described in the opening chapter of this book, there are individuals who desire only natural therapeutics to treat their cancers. While the practitioner should be open-minded to the wishes of the patient, I unfortunately must say that in my practice as a board-certified internist; oncologist; hematologist; nutritionist; geriatrician; and holistic, sports-, integrative-, and complementary-medicine physician, I have *not seen many aggressive and/ or late-stage cancers successfully treated by commonly utilized natural alternative treatments alone.* I have been utilizing an alternative but not natural therapy, as explained below, called Insulin Potentiation Therapy (IPT), and obtaining favorable result for several years.

This is why I went to medical school, did a three-year residency in internal medicine, another three in hematology and oncology, and became board certified in all three (as well as other medical specialties as mentioned above). I did this because I wanted to help patients survive, since I would have other therapies in addition to natural ones to offer when appropriate. I believe you never graduate from the "university of learning"!

The patient should not be blinded by dogma, misinformation, or unfounded hope in a particular treatment, especially if it dissuades the use of others. Do not be fooled by what I call "trick-or-treat" therapies! Sometimes patients with cancer just don't realize the seriousness of the situation!

Cancer kills you if you let it!

Some say, "I feel too well for this to be that serious" and don't take appropriate action. The reasons people do not utilize the most effective treatments are discussed in detail in chapter 12.

Remember, you typically don't "feel it" until you crash, and by that time it's often too late for a cure.

The goal should be *surviving* and being comfortable (quality and quantity)!

Recently I had the opportunity to do a consultation on a thirty-six-year-old mother of two who noted a breast lump, which turned out to be malignant. She refused to remove the cancer surgically and refused all traditional therapies. The cancer had spread to her lungs and the vertebra in her back. She was told she needed emergency radiation to her spine and high doses of steroids (decadron, which is in the prednisone family). She presented to my office to discuss possible alternative therapies.

While I would have liked to honor her wishes about natural therapies, this was a situation where she needed *emergency* radiation to her spine or she would become paralyzed from the waist down and not have control of her bowels or bladder.

When I conveyed this to her and described the poor prognosis associated with withholding treatment, she reluctantly agreed to proceed with the radiation treatments. I assured her we could utilize alternative therapeutics to augment and buffer the side effects of the conventional treatments.

Insulin Potentiation Therapy (IPT) can be an option for treating some cancers. The cell environment in the body can have an effect on cancer. Glucose is a simple sugar in the body appears that plays an important role in cancer growth. The *New York Times* featured an article by Gary Taubes on April 13, 2011. The article reveals that, astoundingly, in western Antarctica, there were only two case of breast cancer between 1967 and 1980. When their diet changed to one similar to a Western diet, the incident of breast cancer dramatically increased. There was a direct correlation between the increase of sugar and the dramatic increase of cancer!

One diagnostic test used for cancer detection is a radiological test called a PET (Positron Emission Tomography) scan. It is used to diagnose cancer and monitor treatment. The study uses FDG (florodeoxyglucose) as a tracer to image cancer cells. Cancer cells have a high affinity for picking up this glucose molecule much more so than normal cells of the body. Therefore, tracking the glucose uptake can locate the cancer.

Insulin opens up cell membranes to take in glucose and other substances. As a result, cells become more metabolically active. Metabolically active cells are more susceptible to chemotherapy. Studies have shown that cancer cells produce more insulin receptors than healthy cells. Breast cancer cells have several times more insulin receptor sites than normal cells.

In the *European Journal of Oncology* article by Alabaster, O., it stated that metabolic modification by insulin enhances methotrexate (a commonly used chemotherapeutic agent) cytotoxicity in MCF-7 human breast cancer cells. It was also stated that *insulin utilized with methotrexate could possibly increase ten-thousand-fold the cytotoxic effect!*

Also see: Pavelic, K. "Correlation of Substances Immunologically Cross-Reactive with Insulin, Glucose, and Growth Hormone in Hodgkin's Lymphoma Patients." *Cancer Lett.* 17 (1982): 81–6.

Schilsky, R. "Characteristics of Membrane Transport of Methotrexate by Cultured Human Breast Cancer Cells." *Biochemistry Pharmacology* 30 (1981): 1537–42.

Gross, G. "Pertubalation by Insulin of Human Breast Cancer Cell Kinetics." *Cancer Research* 44 (1984): 3570–75.

IPT is based on this premise and utilizes chemotherapy along with glucose and insulin to get into and damage the cancer cells more selectively and effectively. First, insulin is administered by an experienced nurse in a *safe and controlled environment* (several glucose levels are taken). Then the chemotherapy and other chosen substances are given, followed by glucose.

This techique targets the cancer cells to selectively take in the chemotherapy and whatever other agents used! As stated above, cancer cells have more insulin receptors; therefore insulin should open the doors into the cancer cell for the chemotherapy. Then chemo is given followed by glucose (as a "chaser"), since cancer avidly consumes it. This pushes the medicines into the cells. The medicines are selectively sandwiched into the cancer cells.

This selectively increases the delivery of medicines into the cancer cells, therefore increasing efficacy and decreasing side effects. *Lower doses of chemo are typically utilized but at an increased frequency.* It is felt that since the cancer cells are better targeted with IPT, lower doses can be as effective if not more so than the conventional chemotherapy infusions delivery methods. Because of this, less side effects are seen with IPT. There is an ongoing clinical study regarding IPT and quality of life.

I am planning to use, when appropriate, conventional chemotherapy protocols and dosing with the IPT delivery technique. This would be capturing the best of both worlds for some patients! This would also be an important and needed study.

Conventional chemotherapy has utilized one aspect of IPT. That is low intensity (dose of chemotherapy) and increasing density (frequency of administering chemotherapy). Rituximab has been proven very effective treating several types of cancers. On p. 571 of the American Society of Hematology Self-Assessment Program, fourth edition, it is recommended to administer rituximab in a divided three-times-a-week schedule. This is recommended in order to reduce possible life-threatening side effects of this frequently utilized and potentially effective medication.

Some conventional physicians ridicule IPT without a full understanding of it. They call it dangerous because blood sugar is lowered with insulin. There are millions of patients who use insulin on a daily basis for diabetes! It is administered via a well-established, safe protocol by trained and experienced nurses. The chemotherapeutic agents used to treat cancer have more potential dangerous side effects than the IPT!

Another misconception is that the typical doses given in ITP are "so small they couldn't be effective." Typically 10 percent of the standard dose (sometimes we give higher doses) is given two times per week for the first and sometimes second month of treatment. Simple math is that at the end of the month, 80 percent of the standard dose is given. Therefore, this also is not an issue.

IPT shouldn't be used for all cancers. There are cancers that can be treated by conventional therapies with a high success rate and a low side-effect profile. ITP should be considered when there isn't an effective traditional chemotherapeutic protocol available or when the patient is end-stage and wants to extend survival time without being debilitated from aggressive, traditional chemotherapy.

Books I found to be well referenced and enable patients and doctors to better understand IPT:

Hauser, Ross A., MD. *Cancer: Treating Cancer with Insulin Potentiation Therapy.*

Ayre, Steven G., MD et al. *The Kinder, Gentler Cancer Treatment: Insulin Potentiation Targeted LowDose™ Therapy.*

The logical assumption would be that a glucose-restricted diet would result in an environment that does not favor the production of cancer cells. *A diet low in sugar is recommended for all, especially cancer patients.*

We also utilize other interesting tools in our quest to kill cancer. There are companies in the United States (Bio-reference) that perform studies called "cell search." They analyze your blood, looking for circulating cancer cells.

Also in the states, Caris Labs can take the original biopsy (or if it is maintained in paraffin) and test various chemotherapeutic agents to see which would be the most effective to kill or slow down the cancer cells. Finally this approach to select chemotherapy (chemosensitivity test) has been accepted, and insurance companies pay for it, in the United States!

Blood can be sent to Greece or Germany (we call them the Greek or the German test), and if cancer cells are in circulation, they are tested to see which chemotherapeutic agents and natural substances may slow down or kill the cancer cells. There are many drugs that have not been tried for many types of cancer. The tests above offer more options when effective conventional treatments are not available. There are drugs that are used for colon cancer but were never tested on lung cancer. When these drugs are used for lung cancer we call this off-protocol or off-label.

The Greek test also analyzes natural substances to see which will be effective or ineffective in slowing down or killing the cancer cells. If you research online you will see many thing touted as being effective at killing cancer. You will not know which to take and will be very confused. This study will enable you to select in a more scientific fashion effective natural substances.

Controlled amino acid therapy (CAAT) is another interesting natural way of fighting cancer. Cancer cells need certain amino acids to multiply and survive. This diet, in short, controls which amino acids you consume. Most of the amino acids you eat are in capsule or powder form. Your diet is also modified in other ways to eliminate other nutrients required for cancer cell growth and replication. Therefore, you starve the cancer cells of their building blocks, and they can no longer multiply. I saw this method used solely in a patient with pancreatic cancer. She outlived her prognosis by two and a half years. Unfortunately she gave up the diet and eventually the disease came back with a vengeance, and she passed on. I still care for her family. When they come for a visit they always say, "If only she kept up with the diet, she'd be alive!"

For more information on the CAAT diet and how to order the controlled amino acids, visit my website or call the office 631-361-6160.

Alternative practitioners measure levels of heavy metals and other toxins in the body, as there are strong links to cancer and other illnesses. Inflammation is now accepted as one of the possible causes of cancer. Heavy metals in the body can cause inflammation. Some of these of substances include aluminum, mercury, nickel, benzene, PCBs, pesticides, herbicides, and others. Once diagnosed, they should be treated. "Chelation" is a process in which heavy metals are flushed away from the bloodstream and body tissues by means of a "chelator" that binds heavy metal ions. They are typically used in cases of mercury or lead poisoning.

It is important to note that high levels of heavy metals are typically picked up when screening otherwise healthy asymptomatic individuals. In my own practice on Long Island, New York, I have surprised many patients by uncovering high aluminum and mercury levels. Some mercury levels have been reported as being so high that the Department of Health will contact the patient!

Think about the products we use on a daily basis in our own homes. Aluminum, which has been linked to higher incidences of dementia, is present in the vast majority of deodorant/antiperspirants that we use on a daily basis and apply directly to our skin. We cook in pots and pans made of aluminum and bring our leftovers from the restaurant home in aluminum foil. Recently, one of my patients proudly showed me an "organic"-labeled juice pack like the kind we would put in our kids' lunchboxes every day. To her surprise, the inside of the box where the juice was stored was lined with aluminum!

The pH of the body, a reflection of how acidic the body is, can have a large impact. Cancer cells thrive in an acidic environment. Acidity can be determined by testing blood, urine, and saliva. Alternative treatments attempt to create a more alkaline or basic environment in the hopes that the growth of cancer cells will be arrested. This can be achieved through a diet rich in leafy green vegetables and low in red meat, with plenty of water intake.

Nutraceuticals (isolated and/or combinations of specific nutrients designed for a specific physiological response) may also impact the rate of cancer growth. There are many examples of how nutrients can alter the cancer process. For example, folate and B12 can reverse the incidence of atypical cells that can convert to cancer. Selenium can reverse precancerous mouth lesions.

However, recent studies have found that people who were taking *high dosages* of folate and beta-carotene supplementation had increased cancers (most commonly lung). The lesson to be learned is that *too much can be as bad as too little.* I get blood tests for B12, folate, selenium, carotene, and other vitamins and/or minerals when indicated. Basing your supplement intake on blood test findings is a scientific approach that should be used to avoid negative results.

Beta carotene, vitamin A, and vitamin E can reverse premalignant plaques, called leukoplakia, in the mouth. Vitamins A, C, and E have been shown to reverse colorectal adenomas (benign polyps that may become malignant). Vitamin E can reverse benign breast disease such as fibrocystic breast disease. Again, I recommend blood tests be done to guide the dosing of these supplements, since *too much can be as bad as too little.*

Vitamin D

According to a 2009 article in *The American Journal of Medicine*, vitamin D has been found to play a vital role in health, and not just in improving bone density. According to this study, low levels of vitamin D can increase your chances of developing all forms of cancer, diabetes, heart attacks, multiple sclerosis, vascular calcifications, rheumatoid arthritis, decreased cognition (brain function), depression, sarcopenia (muscle wasting), and seasonal affective disorders.

The article further states that vitamin D "has the potential to regulate up to two hundred genes to facilitate cell growth and differentiation, and to possibly decrease the risk of cell transformation into a malignant state." In other words, it decreases normal cells from changing into cancer cells. It was also stated that vitamin D receptors were present in most tissues and cells in the body, thus making vitamin D one of the most potent regulators of cellular growth in both normal and cancer cells!

Life Extension magazine has published many articles about vitamin D. They were ahead of the curve. They, like me, do not wait until "the writing is on the wall" to utilize what is obvious and safe. In January 2010, they published an excellent article: "Startling Findings About Vitamin D Levels in Life Extension® Members" by William Faloon. To view this article: http://www. lef.org/magazine/mag2010/jan2010_Startling-Findings-About-Vitamin-D-Levels-in-Life-Extension-Members_01.htm.

There are many examples where diet can either be preventative or causative in cancer. It is the feeling of the author that vegetarians have less cancer and heart disease. It is hard to isolate vegetarianism as a factor in lowering disease, since there are different types of vegetarians; also playing a role are the duration a person is a vegetarian, genetics, and other lifestyle variables.

Diets low in fiber and high in animal protein, fat, and refined carbohydrates are risk factors for colon cancer. Men with prostate diseases, such as enlargement of the prostate or cancer of the prostate, should follow diets that are low in fat, red meat, processed food, simple sugar, and cholesterol because these foods can be causative in nature.

Natural therapeutics that have been prescribed to treat diseases of the prostate, including cancer, include taking the supplements lycopene, saw palmetto, selenium, and bee pollen, as well as drinking phytonutrient-rich green and black tea.

Of course, in diseases of the prostate, hormonal balance is necessary. Male hormone deficiencies and replacement therapies will be discussed in a subsequent chapter.

What is important to stress with diet and nutraceuticals is that while the role in curing an existing cancer may be limited, they play a large and successful role in prevention. These days, there is much public awareness regarding what actually goes into the foods we eat. The August 31, 2009, *Time* magazine cover story is called "The Real Cost of Cheap Food." I encourage you to read it. (Visit their website to obtain a copy.) It discusses the cost/benefit analysis of organic/chemical-free food as compared to conventionally grown crops using pesticides, and meat containing antibiotics and artificial hormones.

The immune system plays an important role in the surveillance of cancers. The practitioner can order lab work to determine whether the immune system is working optimally. If not, there are several ways to enhance it. First, basic health guidelines discussed previously are important (e.g., good nutrition, adequate water intake, rest, sleep, and minimal stress). Substances such as zinc, mushroom, and herbal extracts can naturally enhance the immune response. Hyperthermia (high temperatures) has also been used to augment the response.

Typically, an integrative approach utilizes several methods to combat cancer. This makes it difficult if not impossible to run a controlled statistical medical study, because one would not be able to prove that treatment "x, y, or z" was effective or ineffective, since they were utilized at the same time.

Doctors and patients want the best results possible. This is why the vast majority combine several treatment modalities for the best possible results. Therefore and again it would be very difficult if not impossible to perform a medically acceptable study.

On the other side of the coin, the problem exists that when a new drug is introduced in a clinical trial, there will likely be a *"control arm," where a patient might literally be taking a sugar pill.* People with cancer have a difficult time enrolling in such a trial for obvious reasons, including time constraints. *If it's a "matter of life and death," you don't want to be treated with a placebo.*

In summary, conventional and alternative treatments can be used in a balanced fashion to treat existing cancers and other diseases and to prevent them from developing. The degree to which each modality is used is dependent on the clinical situation, the patient, and treating practitioner.

CHAPTER 7
ANTIAGING MEDICINE

"You don't have to live with it!"

Mr. Smith is a fifty-four-year-old man who goes to his internist because he "doesn't feel right." He tells the doctor that when he was in his twenties, he worked out three times a week for two to three hours at a time. He did four to five sets of each exercise, which included flat and incline bench presses, presses behind the neck, triceps extensions, barbell and dumbbell curls, lat pull downs, squats, sit ups, leg raises, and other exercises. Mr. Smith stated that when he was in his thirties, he decreased to two to three sets and worked out two to three times per week. In his forties, he went down to one or two sets and worked out two times per week.

Now in his fifties, he does one set and works out one or two times per week. His maximum lifts have decreased dramatically; where he could in the past bench 255 pounds, he can now only do 190. He also feels that his energy and concentration have decreased, he has been putting on weight, and he finds new facial wrinkles every month or so.

He was also concerned because his libido, erections, and sexual activity had markedly decreased. Approximately a year ago, he was sexually active three to four times per week and was now down to one or two times per month. These realizations also contribute to his feelings of depression and hopelessness.

The January 15, 2010, article, "Sexual Activity, Erectile Dysfunction, and Incident Cardiovascular Events," published in *The American Journal of Cardiology* concluded that "low frequency of sexual activity predicts cardiovascular disease independently of erectile dysfunction and that screening for sexual activity might be clinically useful."

The doctor examines Mr. Smith thoroughly and orders blood work to test for anemia, low thyroid, and electrolyte abnormalities, in addition to an electrocardiogram. Mr. Smith returns to the doctor's office in ten days to discuss the results of his tests. The doctor tells Mr. Smith that the examination and all other tests were normal and reassures him. Mr. Smith asks the doctor, "Why are all these things happening to me?" The doctor replies, "You're getting older." Mr. Smith leaves the office not with a sense of reassurance but feeling anxious, defeated, and helpless.

I do not accept statements such as, "You're not as young as you used to be," "You'll have to live with it," or "Dying of natural causes." Are we destined to accept the "inevitable" aging process without a fight? Do we come into this world preprogrammed to deteriorate and die within a certain timeframe, or can our genetics be modified to live longer and healthier lives?

Antiaging medicine and current medical practices are attempting to increase life span and improve the quality of human life. They attempt to increase the individual's "health span" (years spent in good health). Antiaging medicine as a specialty tends to be more proactive and utilizes cutting-edge approaches.

As we age, multiple hormone abnormalities develop in the body and can be diagnosed clinically through extensive specialized lab work. These abnormalities, typically deficiencies, can cause weakness, fatigue, loss of libido, and decreased ambition and productivity. Growth hormone deficiencies are diagnosed through blood work. Growth hormone is important for both the young and old. It should be considered a maintenance hormone. It helps maintain muscle mass and energy, stimulates the incorporation of amino acids into muscle and other organs and tissues, and decreases body fat. It also has many other important functions involving several different cell types of the body.

Beginning in your late twenties, human growth hormone secretion declines about 14 percent per decade. By age sixty, you only secrete 25 percent as much growth hormone as an average twenty-year-old. This growth hormone reduction greatly contributes to the aging process. If there is a true deficiency, I will first utilize various natural supplements (usually without injections), and then reevaluate the patient clinically, and with blood tests. Only when natural products fail to elevate growth hormone levels into the normal range do use injections of it.

In my antiaging medicine practice, specific emphasis is placed on menopause in females and andropause in males. In women, natural therapeutics and bioidentical hormones (hormones that are "identical" on a molecular level with hormones the body naturally produces), as opposed to synthetic hormones, are used to increase the "good" estrogen and decrease the potentially carcinogenic (cancer-causing) "bad" estrogens. While most have heard of female menopause, few have heard of the real syndrome of male menopause.

In fact, I have done extensive lecturing on both topics and have found more interest by men in coming to these talks than women. This is perhaps because few medical practitioners discuss this topic with their male patients either due to their lack of knowledge or from pure discomfort.

In men, clinical deficiencies in testosterone or its precursors or situations in which testosterone deficiencies arise from age-related conversion or testosterone to estrogen are treated with natural therapeutics. Only when all natural attempts to correct laboratory and clinical abnormalities have failed will other therapies be utilized (e.g., gels, creams, injections).

The decrease in hormones as we age has simply been called hormonal "pauses." Science has now documented that several important anabolic (body-building) hormones decrease in a predictable fashion as we get older:

❖ Decreased DHEA

❖ Decreased total testosterone

❖ Decreased free testosterone

❖ Decreased growth hormone

❖ Decreased estrogen and progesterone

❖ Decreased IGF-1 (insulin-like growth factor)

It is primarily the decrease in testosterone that causes male menopause, and the decrease in estrogen and progesterone that causes female menopause. The symptoms of female menopause include decreased libido, decreased vaginal lubrication and breast tone, weight gain, and hair loss.

Symptoms of male menopause include weakness, fatigue, loss of libido, and impotence. The goal of hormone replacement therapy is to alleviate these symptoms and to help promote overall increased health, life span, and a sense of well-being. Visit Life Extension's website (see reference/bibliography section) for many terrific articles covering male and female menopause.

Women who enter menopause are often plagued by a variety of symptoms, such as hot flashes ("power surges," as a friend calls them), weight gain, decreased libido, anxiety, depression, and difficulty sleeping. After first convincing themselves they are not losing their sanity, they often visit their gynecologist to seek help with these symptoms. Often they are started on hormones. Standard hormone replacement in women is prescribed utilizing hormones obtained from the urine of pregnant horses (i.e., premarin: pregnant mares' urine), a less-than-pleasant thought, particularly with my patients who are vegetarians.

For treatment of symptomatic hormone deficiency in women, our practice utilizes bio identical hormones. These are nonsynthetic hormones derived from soy and yams. They are what I consider to be bio-similar in chemical structure to hormones that are produced naturally by a women.

Testosterone is important for females as well and helps with energy, strength, bone density, libido, fat metabolism, skin wrinkling, and an overall sense of well-being. The Mayo Clinic included a special supplement to their journal on April 2004 that was devoted to androgen (testosterone) therapy for females. Levels of total and free testosterone, along with other hormones mentioned should be tested to determine the cause of low levels of testosterone. The cause, if found, should be treated. I have had an approximately 85 percent success rate in elevating testosterone levels without using actual testosterone preparations. Prior to initiating treatment in our office, the patient is sent for an extensive blood hormone assay, as there are several different hormones involved in the estrogen and testosterone hormonal cascade. This must be done so the cause of any deficiency and/or any imbalances can be identified and treated appropriately. *The cure is in the cause!*

It is also common medical practice to treat patients in a one-size-fits-all fashion. For example, a ninety-three-pound woman is likely to receive the same dose of estrogen as a two-hundred-pound woman. Once we have determined the patient's needs based on her degree of hormone deficiency, weight, and other individualized parameters, a prescription is sent to a "compounding pharmacy," which will then compound the correct "personalized" prescription for the patient.

The patient is subsequently reevaluated clinically and via blood work to determine the response to the prescription. In addition to bio identical hormonal replacement, lifestyle modification and supplementation is utilized.

In men, deficiencies of male sex hormones may occur at different levels, from the central axis of the pituitary and the hypothalamus of the brain to the level of the testicles. The pituitary gland may be working overtime, but if there is a failure of the testicles to respond and make testosterone, there will be a true deficiency. HRT must therefore target the presumed fail point in this complicated pathway.

Treatment plans may include replacing testosterone; replacing DHEA (which is a precursor molecule for testosterone); blocking conversion in the body of testosterone to estrogen; and others. It must be noted that determining whether a man is deficient in testosterone is difficult to interpret with only basic lab work. *The cure of low testosterone is in the cause.*

The normal range of testosterone in the blood varies greatly. Let's say, for example, that a man in his sixties presents to our office with fatigue, muscle weakness, and loss of libido. We do a blood testosterone level and it comes back two hundred. Is this number low for this patient? Are his symptoms attributable to this level? Is he in male menopause?

The answer depends in part on the patient's baseline level when he was younger. If we had the luxury of measuring this patient's testosterone when he was in his thirties, we might have found the level to be nine hundred. If so, his current level of two hundred is significantly lower, and this relative drop might cause his symptoms. If, however, his prior level was three hundred, this drop is less significant.

A baseline test is obviously an important step toward a man's overall health assessment. In my practice, I perform a "preaging" screening in younger patients to establish baseline levels of many hormones. This will help identify what is normal for the patient at a young age such that we can utilize this information as a comparison in years to come. I cannot stress enough that every patient has his or her own set point dictated by DNA and environment, and every patient must be treated as a unique individual when devising a treatment plan.

Not every patient is a candidate for hormone replacement. Women with a personal or family history of breast issues, men with prostate cancer that has not been treated definitively (removed), a personal or family history of deep-vein thrombosis or pulmonary embolisms (clots), and other situations that are beyond the scope of this book I would not treat with hormone replacement. For more information call the office at 631-361-6160 or visit our website: www.agingalternative.com.

In addition to some of the specifics outlined above, our antiaging practice stresses the importance of proper nutrition, exercise, rest, and preventive care. The ultimate goal is to facilitate "healthy aging." The organization called Life Extension has many high-quality, cutting-edge products that I recommend to promote longevity. I recommend and personally take CR Mimmicer, Apple Wise, Carnosine, CoQ10, and PQQ.

> *You're never too old to become younger.*
> —Mae West

CHAPTER 8
OBESITY

Two-thirds of adults in the United States are considered overweight. About a third of these are considered obese. Obesity is defined as excess body fat—greater than 25 percent in females and 20 percent in males. It can also be defined as a body mass index (BMI: weight in pounds divided by height in inches squared times 703) greater than 25 percent. Among children between six and nineteen years of age, 15 percent—one in six—are overweight. People always seem to make a fuss over the adorable chubby baby. In actuality, the excess weight is not only creating bad eating dynamics from the start, but forms the beginnings of cholesterol streaks that deposit in arteries even at age two or three.

Clearly these numbers are significant and are increasing. Even more than 25 percent of our dogs and cats are overweight, so we are passing our bad habits on to them. Why is obesity such an important health issue? Obesity is a major concern since it affects adults, children, and pets worldwide.

It is known that obesity causes increased risk of diabetes, hypertension, heart disease, abnormal cholesterol profile, cancer, sleep apnea, and back, knee, and joint pain. It is common for a patient to present to his or her doctor for a checkup and routine blood work, which may reveal elevated blood glucose. The patient may truly have diabetes and require treatment with oral medications or insulin shots; however, a certain population of individuals who are obese may show improvement in their fasting blood sugar levels if they lose a significant amount of weight and change their lifestyle. They may be able to eliminate or delay the need for medications, therefore lessening diabetic complications such as heart and peripheral vascular disease, kidney failure, and infections.

Several years ago, a study published in *Emergency Medicine* reported that the risk of death from cancer is 52 percent higher for obese men and 62 percent higher for obese women than people of normal weights.

It has also been documented that calorie restriction can prolong life span. Obesity has been linked with many different types of cancers, including breast, uterine, colon, liver, gallbladder, pancreas, stomach, and prostate. In addition to medical complications of obesity, psychosocial issues should be considered. In a society that idolizes five-feet-ten-inch female models who wear a size zero, being obese can cause significant depression and a sense of worthlessness. It can even lead to psychological eating disorders such as bulimia and anorexia.

Why are so many Americans overweight? The reasons are multifactorial. First, some individuals are genetically programmed to be overweight. There are metabolic disorders that can lead to obesity, such as hypothyroidism (a deficiency of thyroid hormone), low testosterone, menopause, diabetes, growth hormone deficiency, etc. Consultation with your doctor to include a detailed physical and blood work can rule out many medical disorders.

In some cases, obesity may be sociocultural, as certain populations are clearly more likely to be obese than others. There are psychological reasons why people overeat or eat incorrectly. Some people eat when they are under stress, because it brings them into some type of a comfort zone; it makes them feel better. Other people look at food as a reward at the end of the day after they have worked hard.

It is important for the practitioner to delve into these issues because they may be correctable. Sometimes referral for psychological counseling may be helpful. The hardest part for the patient is to admit there is a problem that can lead to significant health risk, but with hard work it can be correctable. It is notable that we are discussing obesity in the United States. Other countries such as Japan do not have this same problem with obesity. Is overeating genetic, learned behavior, or a combination of both?

However, the overwhelming majority of people who are overweight are this way because they simply eat too much of the wrong foods and don't exercise enough. While most people would prefer not to be overweight or unhealthy, the fast-food industry makes this very difficult. With an increasingly busy work schedule for most people, there is less time for food shopping and preparation. The multitude of available fast-food restaurants and processed food preparations provides an easy, inexpensive, and often extremely unhealthy option.

An article by Gary Taubes in the *New York Times* in April 13, 2011, showed a direct correlation to sugar and cancer. The article stated that the average American eats about ninety pounds of sugar a year!

There are simple changes in your eating habits that can help you lose weight. Here are a few.

- Use smaller plates and dishes.

- Cut food into small pieces.

- Eat one piece at a time.

- While chewing, put down your fork or spoon between bites.

- Chew all food thoroughly and enjoy the taste.

- Do not talk while eating.

- Give yourself more work while eating. Eat the peanuts that have to be removed from the shells rather than the shelled peanuts, and you will be guaranteed to eat less.

- Eat the right kinds (healthy, natural, colorful) of unprocessed foods.

- Eat slowly.

- Stop when you are getting full; do not overeat.

- Eat smaller meals more frequently.

- Avoid eating at least three hours before you go to bed or prolonged relaxation, as what you eat will not be properly digested and more likely to be converted to a storage form energy such as glycogen and/or fat since it will not be utilized for energy. Literally your body goes into hibernation when sleeping or resting and stores food as fat!

Now that we have discussed what not to eat, we must ask, what should we eat? In general, the healthiest diets are those that are lowest in fat, calories, carbohydrates, and sugars and should be low in quantities of red meat. The diet should be "high density"—foods that fill you up without adding calories—including grains, vegetables, and fruits.

Vegetarian diets are healthy as long as a sufficient amount of protein is obtained from nuts, seeds, and soy. (Living on potato chips is not considered a healthy "vegetarian" diet!) Vegetarians can be prone to developing protein, vitamin B, and other deficiencies. This is why appropriate blood testing should be periodically performed by a physician familiar with vegetarian diets.

It is also important to drink eight to ten glasses of pure water per day because it keeps you hydrated and helps cleanse impurities and toxins from your system. Caffeinated and alcoholic beverages in general do not count as they can increase urination and promote loss of water from the body. For more detail go to www.watercure.com.

There are many weight-loss diets that are available and advertised. I would caution you against "diet pills" and programs that cause rapid weight loss. A slow but sure weight loss is better than a quick-results starvation diet. Not only is slow weight loss healthier to your system, it enables you to modify and learn new and improved eating and exercise habits for a lifetime.

A quick weight loss will likely result in a rebound effect, returning you to your original weight—or worse, even heavier than the weight you started from. You should sit down with your doctor and establish reasonable short- and long-term goals for your weight-loss efforts. Try working with your spouse or a friend so that you can give each other moral support and feel that you are not alone.

The benefits of exercise cannot be stressed enough. Besides aiding in weight loss, exercise itself offers many long-term benefits to your health, including improving cardiovascular and pulmonary function and improving your sense of well-being.

Combining aerobic exercise with weight training as opposed to aerobic exercise alone may be the best way to lose weight and achieve overall health and fitness. Thirty-five-hundred calories burned equals one pound of weight lost. The following is a list of activities and the calories expended per hour for a typical 150-pound person:

- Lying at ease: 90 calories

- Walking three mph: 300 calories

- Running an eleven-   520 calories
  and-a-half-minute mile:

- Running an eight-minute mile: 852 calories

- Rowing machine: 486 calories

- Swimming slowly: 520 calories

- Tennis: 444 calories

- Golf: 348 calories

- Horseback riding: 450 calories

In addition to diet, exercise, and behavioral modification, alternative practitioners may recommend some natural products to aid in weight loss.

Some obese individuals are, for a variety of reasons, unable to lose weight under any prescribed method. If many different approaches have been tried and failed, bariatric surgery may be the answer. Simply put, this type of surgery attempts to surgically minimize the amount of food that can be ingested by the individual. Often this is done by physically making the stomach smaller; therefore, you are not able to eat as much and you feel fuller much quicker. Absorption of food is also decreased, therefore taking in fewer calories. Bariatric surgery, however, is not a "total cure" and can result in nutritional deficiencies and other complications.

It has been my experience that people who have the surgery feel they can eat any type of food that they want if they cut down on portions. It is still important to modify your diet after the surgery and eat healthy low-fat, low-calorie food. The "sweet syndrome" is when one eats sweets like ice cream, which is absorbed in spite of the surgery. This unfortunately "outsmarts" the bariatric surgery, and they gain weight back! This is why one must look into all possible options, benefits, and side effects prior to any medical or surgical decision.

Mainstream medicine is actively addressing the widespread problem of obesity. However, due to time constraints, most physicians do not have the time to work out an individualized, detailed plan of weight management with the patient. Sometimes drugs are prescribed for weight loss. Again, one must look into all possible options, benefits, and side effects prior to any medical decision.

Complementary/integrative practitioners are able to put more time and emphasis on developing individualized strategies utilizing diet and exercise programs in addition to such modalities as nutraceuticals, acupuncture, hypnosis, and psychological counseling. They may also refer a patient to a nutritionist and other specialists for further help.

CHAPTER 9
TOXIC SOLUTIONS

On a recent occasion, one of my patients brought in his teenage daughter so I could render an opinion on her condition. She had what I would medically consider a mild case of acne. However, this was causing her great distress. She went to a general practitioner, not a dermatologist, who evaluated her and recommended that she start on a medicine that would likely improve her acne.

However, this particular medication required the patient to sign a disclaimer stating she understood and accepted certain side effects and risks before she would be given a prescription. The side effects included liver damage, altered and aggressive behavior, depression and suicide, hearing impairment, cataracts, seizure, stroke, bone marrow suppression, and severe potential toxicities to a fetus should pregnancy occur.

Naturally the contents of this form were disconcerting to my patient and his daughter, and they were hesitant to start the medication. I informed the patient that long-term use of this medication has shown it to be effective in treating severe cases of acne; however, in my opinion, the *side effect/risk profile was unacceptable* for someone with mild acne. This brings up an important concept. The treatment should be commensurate with the disease or condition. The benefits should, of course, outweigh the side effects. You don't want to win a battle and lose the war. A famous phrase physicians live by is "Do no harm."

When a life-threatening illness such as metastatic cancer is diagnosed, treatments that have potentially toxic side effects may be the course to take. We know that chemotherapy can cause a wide variety of side effects such as suppression of the bone marrow, nausea, vomiting, infection, hair loss, and liver, kidney, and cardiac damage. However, treatment can be lifesaving, and therefore, the risks can be justified.

Doctors often end up in difficult positions where they have patients with terminal illnesses willing to try experimental medications that may prolong their lives but may also make them worse symptomatically. In this situation, one should be aware of the possible side effects but hopefully still take advantage of the benefits. Clearly, life-threatening risks would not be utilized for lesser conditions that have proven and less toxic treatments available.

In critical situations in the emergency room, doctors wrestle with this dilemma. They must determine the risk/benefit ratio of their actions to maximize good and minimize bad outcomes. The hospital I work for is a center for emergency cardiac catheterization, angioplasty, and stent placement, as well as a stroke center. When patients present with a heart attack or a stroke, they may be candidates for either invasive cardiac testing, interventions, or clot-busting medication, respectively. How is the determination made as to how to proceed? A benefit-versus-side-effects analysis is quickly performed by the physician.

There is always a small risk of a negative outcome in which the patient will get worse. When patients present early on with a heart attack or stroke, we know there is a high likelihood that we can make them better with a small risk. If they present later on, the likelihood of improvement is lesser. Thus, over time, the likelihood of improvement approaches the likelihood of a negative outcome, and the risk is no longer acceptable. Therefore if you procrastinate, lifesaving procedures and medicines that could have helped cannot be used.

Certain patients are intrinsically high risks because of bleeding disorders, very old age, or other comorbid factors (diabetes, heart, lung, liver, kidney diseases). This must be taken into consideration at all times when treating patients.

With regard to my patient whose daughter had the acne, I presented another treatment approach. First we sent off blood work, which revealed the patient to have an elevated aluminum level in her blood, and her estrone (an estrogenic hormone secreted by the ovary and fatty tissue that if elevated can cause cancer) level was also elevated. Her diet was very unhealthy. It included much too much fried, fast, and other junk food.

We treated her elevated estrone and aluminum with natural products. We also modified her diet to avoid junk food and increased her intake of water, fruit, and leafy green vegetables. We utilized natural skin cleaner (tea tree soap) and added zinc, fish oil, and acidophilus supplements.

With these interventions, her acne improved 80–90 percent and has remained so for the last two years. More importantly, she is much happier about herself and feels better, healthier, and is more health conscious. As an extra benefit, we have corrected the blood abnormalities we discussed.

Another situation where conventional medicine can perform "overkill" is with treatment of hair loss. There is a group of medicines that cause the blockade of the male hormone dihydrotestosterone (DHT) that is used to treat enlarged prostates and difficulty urinating. Sometimes DHT blockers are prescribed to combat hair loss in men. It did help reverse the hair loss in some of the men I treated for other issues including the side effects from these drugs.

A new patient arrived at my office complaining of sexual dysfunction and loss of libido, which was clearly very disturbing in a thirty-three-year-old male. When interviewing the patient, he informed me that a DHT blocker had been prescribed for him to treat premature hair loss. Sexual malfunction can be a side effect of this medication. We discontinued the medicine and allowed its effects to dissipate. We then drew baseline blood levels of testosterone and its related compounds. The patient was started on various natural supplements, such as saw palmetto.

After approximately two months the blood work was repeated and the DHT level was found to have decreased significantly without the negative side effect of sexual malfunction. In addition, the original goal of slowing hair loss had been achieved. We also used simple measures such as shampoos that washed out completely and did not block the hair follicles, and changing positions during sleep, as lying in the same position can cause the hair to be lost from areas of constant direct pressure.

At this point, I must mention a patient in my practice with a troublesome disease that turned out to have a truly gratifying outcome. I recently started caring for a twenty-year-old male who had contracted Lyme disease about seven years ago. Since the time of diagnosis he has been treated with multiple courses of different antibiotics. In spite of appropriate treatment, he continued to experience fatigue, muscle pain, and difficulty concentrating. He had been an A student and now had such severe fatigue and problems concentrating that his grades were suffering. He was feeling depressed and helpless. Out of persistence by his parents he was taken to multiple practitioners, where different treatments were tried. He was treated in a bariatric chamber, sauna baths, and was put on strict diets and received multiple supplements. In spite of this, his symptoms failed to subside.

He was brought in to my office by his concerned father. After taking his history and conducting a physical exam, I ordered extensive lab work, including a hormone profile. To my surprise there were multiple hormone deficiencies revealed. Were these deficiencies a result of suppression by a chronic infection? I have seen this phenomenon in other infectious conditions, but at this time I can only say my experience is anecdotal.

Based on the lab work, the patient was started on an oral supplementation to elevate his hormonal deficiencies. Within several weeks he returned to see me. He was like a new person, with more energy and without difficulty concentrating. His repeat blood work showed marked improvement.

I have had several other patients with similar results. Clearly more experience is needed to make any conclusions about treating symptoms of Lyme disease in this manner. But for this patient, and others, they are glad to be back to normal. They also had extensive courses of antibiotics.

I have also found that some patients with Lyme disease require *longer courses of antibiotic* treatments than typically recommended by conventional medicine. However some alternate practitioners recommend two years of uninterrupted intravenous antibiotic. I have not seen this approach be beneficial. Furthermore, this can cause several side effects. Again, *too much can be as bad as too little!*

My son noticed he had a large reddish rash on his chest. The next day the left side of his face and neck was not moving! Lumbar puncture was positive for Lyme disease. He received twenty-one days of intravenous antibiotics, and I gave him several herbs, intravenous supplementation, and nutraceuticals. I have also given him oral antibiotic when his left eyelid appears to be lower than the right. So far he has been asymptomatic for more than a year.

If you think you have Lyme disease see a physician who utilizes a lab that tests for several strains of Lyme, or else the diagnosis could be missed. A longer course of varied antibiotics and several alternative therapies should be utilized in order to eradicate the three major forms of the disease.

CHAPTER 10

COMMON DRUG AND SUPPLEMENT MISTAKES/INTERACTIONS

There are many patients who take numerous medications—patients in my own practice take as many as thirty different medications! Clearly, when taking so many medications, there is the potential for interactions and side effects.

A patient of mine said, "They're making up new syndromes and diseases so they can invent new drugs." The same patient added, "It seems we have a pill for every ill."

Another said it seemed as if "medicine has become a pill-and-bill machine."

Recently aired on CNN several concerns were discussed regarding children and young adults being placed on multiple psychotropic medications.

I think the reason we are such a well-medicated society is not just due the current practice of medicine. It is much more complicated and multifaceted. It could also be attributed to family, economic, social, and medical legal issues. Be that as it may, taking multiple medications can lead to possible complications.

Sometimes multiple medications are needed and are potentially life saving. The patient should be mindful and discuss with his or her caretakers all supplements and medications he or she are taking. This includes medical doctors, naturopaths, nutritionists, herbalists, chiropractors, acupuncturists, and other clinicians that may be caring for you or a loved one.

When adding supplements to the medication regimen, additional side effects must be considered. Often, patients add these supplements themselves, or a second practitioner may add them. The primary prescribing physician may be unaware that the patient is taking supplements or may not have the knowledge about supplements to predict potential interactions with the patient's other medicines.

There are many drug and supplement mistakes and interactions. It is beyond the scope of this book to discuss them all. We will discuss the more common and more important ones. When combining both prescription and OTC medications/supplements, one should read all labels, warnings, and interactions, and discuss them with his or her physician.

Common interactions include:

• increasing or decreasing the effectiveness of either the medication or supplement;

• increasing or decreasing the known side effects;

• previously unknown side effects being created by combining the medications; and

- incorrect use of a drug or supplement in a clinical setting (e.g., incorrect dosage, form, or combinations).

Common possible interactions:

Several natural products and drugs can interfere with drug metabolism. This can cause the actual blood level of medication to be too low or high. This is particularly important when patients with cancer are taking chemotherapy medications that are metabolized in the liver:

Cyclophosphamide
Docetaxel
Etoposide
Ifosfamide
Irinotecan
Paclitaxel
Vinblastine
Vincristine
Vinorelbine

Herbals and medications that interfere with an enzyme in the liver called cytochrome P 450 metabolizes (breaks down) medications; therefore, the *drug level increases and can become toxic.*

Common natural substances and drugs that could elevate drug levels include but are not limited to:

Grapefruit juice
Milk thistle
Goldenseal

Cat's claw

Licorice

Chamomile

Wild cherry

Cannabinoids (marijuana)

Danazol

Erythromycin

Biaxin

Zithromax

Ketoconazole

Amiodarone

Chloramphenicol

Diltiazem

Quinine sulfates

Rifampin

Isoniazid

Tamoxifen

Tumor necrosis blocking agents

Vaccines/toxoids

Verapamil

St. John's Wort has been studied in mainstream medicine and found to be effective for mild to moderate depression. However care must be taken when using it with other medications. It can cause several unwanted side effects when combined with the above herbals and medications. It increases the P 450 enzyme in the liver via its major constituent, a substance called hyperforin. This will *decrease the medication and therefore its likelihood of its effectiveness.*

It should be highlighted that St. John's Wort can decrease a commonly used chemotherapeutic agent called irinotecan active metabolite greater than 50 percent. See p. 569 *Cancer Principles & Practice of Oncology Review,* second edition or the textbook *Cancer* by DeVita, Hellman, and Rosenberg for more detail regarding drug interactions.

Common medications that can *decrease drug levels* include but are not limited to:

> Phenobarbital
> Dilantin
> Carbamazepine (tegretol)
> Citalopram (celexa)
> Clozapine
> Digoxin
> Fluoxetine (Prozac)
> Griseofulvins
> Sertraline (Zoloft)
> Trazodone

There are numerous drugs and natural products that can be potentially liver toxic. Again I highly recommend that *you study any drug and/or natural products that you are taking or contemplating tak*ing.

We will now refer to specific examples.

Statin drugs are used extensively to treat high cholesterol and have proven success in treating heart disease. When using a statin drug for elevated cholesterol, one should be aware of the several side effects when used alone and in combination with other drugs, supplements, and food. They can affect muscle tissue, causing pain (myopathy), and when severe can destroy muscle tissue (rhabdomyolysis). The former can be extremely dangerous, and when a patient has muscle pain he or she should immediately call a physician.

Blood testing while on statin drugs and red yeast rice (a natural product used to lower cholesterol) should include: creatine phosphokinase, liver enzymes, CoQ10, and electrolytes. If the bloods test are abnormal, the statin medication and/or the red yeast rice should be halted until a physician determines the next appropriate step.

Hepatoxicity (liver toxicity) should always be considered when there is upper right abdominal pain, nausea, vomiting, and/or skin yellowing. Liver enzyme blood tests should be immediately obtained, and the statin should be stopped until the results are reviewed. Muscle stiffness and joint pain could indicate direct toxicity and the medicine should be discontinued.

Other side effects associated with statin drugs include but are not limited to headaches; rashes (from benign to severe conditions such as erythema multiforme, toxic epidermal necrolysis, and Stevens-Johnson syndrome); infections; kidney failure; lupus; pancreatitis; hypersensitivity reactions; vasculitis (inflammation of blood vessels); polymyalgia rheumatica; tendon rupture; leucopenia (low white blood cells); thrombocytopenia (low platelets); back and abdominal pain; and others.

There are certain well-known interactions with the statin drugs. Statins are contraindicated with azole antifungals and protease inhibitor medications. They should also be avoided with zafirlukast; thiotepa; telithromycin; telbivudine; silodosin; rifampins; red yeast; red clover; ranolazine; quinupristin/dalfopristin; niacin; nefazodone; imatinib; gemfibrozil; fluvoxamine; ezetimibe; erythromycins; delavirdine; cyclosporine; conivaptan; clarithromycins; and danazol. Caution is advised with herbals such as cat's claw; black cohosh; goldenseal; gotu kola; kava; licorice; milk thistle; and St. John's Wort. If you are combining a statin drug with any of the above medicines or natural products, care must be taken! You should go to a practitioner who is familiar with this situation.

Several other drugs should be used cautiously. Some examples are tumor necrosis factor agents (used for cancer, rheumatoid arthritis), oral contraceptives, and chemotherapy; it is important not to consume acidic fruit juice such as grapefruit. The substance bergamottin contained in grapefruit inactivates digestive enzymes that break down statin drugs (and others). This can significantly increase blood level of the statin drug, causing side effects.

Now, understandably, this is a scary list of medications that interact with only one group of drugs. So how can you possibly sort this out? Well, to begin, you must elicit the help of your physician and your local pharmacist, and be your own health advocate.

Does this scary side effect profile mean that no one should take statin drugs? No. Statins are important drugs, but there are three important points to be made. First, you should always speak to your doctor about any potential side effects and warning signs. Second, you should act on any warnings your body gives you and immediately call your doctor. Third, your doctor should be aware of any over-the-counter or practitioner-prescribed products you are taking in order to identify or predict potential problems before they start.

Alternative practitioners primarily use red yeast rice to lower cholesterol. Its mechanism of action is similar to a statin drug's. It could cause similar side effects. I have prescribed it hundreds of times, and one patient who had muscle soreness from a statin drug had the same side effect while taking red yeast rice supplements. Patients on red yeast rice should be followed the same as if they were on statin drugs. This should include regular blood tests and doctor visits.

The January 15, 2010, article "Tolerability of Red Yeast Rice (2,400mg Twice Daily) versus Pravastatin (20mg Twice Daily) in Patients With Previous Statin Intolerance," published in *The American Journal of Cardiology,* found that LDL ("bad" cholesterol) was reduced 30 percent in the red yeast group and 27 percent in the pravastatin group. An impressive 93 percent of the patients who had statin-related muscle pain (myalgia) tolerated red yeast rice. This is important, since muscle symptoms often recur when a different statin is tried.

Several drugs, herbal supplements, and vitamins can cause increased bleeding. They must be used cautiously whether alone or in combination. Some drugs associated with increased bleeding include warfarin; lovenox; aspirin; plavix; nonsteroidal anti-inflammatory medicines (ibuprofen, Advil, naprosyn, indocin, etc.); Cox 2 inhibitors; SSRIs; and alcohol. If you're taking warfarin or aspirin for heart disease, you should not take ibuprofen in addition, for pain. This can cause severe bleeding, most notably in the GI tract, even in small doses.

Several chemotherapeutic agents can cause bleeding, primarily by lowering the platelet count. There are many others drugs that interfere with clotting, so you should check with your PCP or primary clinician before taking any new medication or supplement.

It is also worth mentioning that elderly patients should exercise extreme caution with all medications. As elderly people metabolize medications more slowly due to changes in the kidneys, liver, and volume of fat distribution, the medicines they take may accumulate in the body. This makes them more susceptible to negative side effects from single medications and certainly from combinations of drugs.

A relative of mine who is eighty-seven years young recently underwent orthopedic surgery under general anesthesia and subsequently received narcotic pain medications. The night of the surgery, this sweet man became combative, angry, disoriented, and confused, even striking out against his wife. While he was somewhat better in the morning, the confusion and even hallucinations persisted for several days.

According to orthopedic practitioners I have spoken to, this is quite common after orthopedic surgical procedures in the elderly. Much of the altered behavior can be attributed to toxic accumulation of narcotics, as the elderly are not able to clear medicines from their systems at the same rate as younger individuals. I am happy to say that my relative is home in his own environment and is doing well.

Supplements and herbals that can interfere with clotting include but are not limited to vitamin E, fish oil, flaxseed, garlic, ginger, Ginkgo biloba, glucosamine, goldenseal, green tea, and willow bark (please see the *Physicians Desk Reference* (http://www.pdr.net/), as well as other medical texts, for a complete list).

Since osteoporosis has become "villainous," women have been ingesting calcium pills on a daily basis. Unfortunately, I called the turn thirty or so years ago, predicting that there would be an increase of "hardening of the arteries." You see, hardening of the arteries, or atherosclerosis, isn't just a problem with cholesterol. There is also calcium, clotting factors, and muscle growth within the wall of the artery that can cause the narrowing of the artery. This causes decreased blood flow to the area. This can cause heart attacks, peripheral vascular disease, and strokes.

Indeed, studies have shown an increase in heart disease in women taking calcium tablets. Interestingly, there are studies now that show that if one takes vitamin K2 with their calcium, they may lessen there risk of heart disease. Please review an excellent article in *Life Extension* in their August 2012 issue, titled "How Calcium May Cause Heart Attack" for further information.

My dear patient Mr. Juda kindly allowed me to share his story. He was a bodybuilder and who drank five quarts of milk every day for many years. He came to me at the age of sixty-eight with calcified carotid arteries and valves of his heart, confirmed by sonogram and echocardiogram. He wanted to try a natural approach to remove the calcium. I told him I would try since he was at a critical point, but there were no guarantees. We would also have to be scientific by periodically repeating the sonograms of his heart and carotids to see if we were being effective or if the disease was progressing.

We first used IV chelation therapy—which involves a series of intravenous injections of a binding (chelating) agent to remove toxic metals and wastes from the bloodstream—using EDTA and vitamin C. We reduced his cholesterol markedly with natural supplements and reduced his calcium intake through his diet and other things. After several months of treatment, we repeated the ultrasounds of the carotid arteries and heart valves and did not see much of a change. He wanted to proceed with the natural therapeutic approach. We then used IV K2, phosphatidylcholine, magnesium, glutethione, and other products. We also lowered his cholesterol and LDL with red yeast rice. His HDL was increased with fish oil and niacin. The calcium plaque was attacked with oral magnesium, IP6, and vitamins D and K2.

Repeat ultrasounds showed approximately 30 percent improvement in one of the carotid arteries, but the other that had originally 90 percent blockage worsened. I think it worsened because whatever we used did not adequately get into the artery to remove the calcium since it was so blocked

He was at critical point with the one carotid artery, which was now more than 90 percent blocked and could potentially lead to a stroke. After discussing his options and likely outcomes, he decided at this point to have an endarterectomy (bypass) of that carotid artery. At the time of this writing, he had the procedure three days ago. He is doing well since the surgery. He wants to continue the treatments in order to prevent the bypass from developing plaque and continue to remove calcium from his heart valves and other carotid artery with which we had favorable results.

Several learning points are noted from this case. Patient safety is the most important thing when treating with any modality. This patient was stable and could be treated conservatively. Patients should be followed up closely and in a scientific fashion. If a treatment isn't working, move on and change the approach. Don't stay with a losing horse! When a patient is in a critical situation, appropriate definitive measures should be taken in an urgent fashion.

I have been testing and treating vitamin D deficiencies for several years before it was accepted into mainstream traditional medicine. Vitamin D deficiency *and excess* can both cause vascular calcifications. I am happy that mainstream medicine has recognized the significance of vitamin D, but not totally with the manner it is being treated. It's usually treated with fifty thousand units of vitamin D2. I consider this *industrial strength* treatment for most patients. This approach I feel could be appropriate for severe deficiencies, cancer, and autoimmune diseases.

If you have a true vitamin D deficiency as discussed in the next paragraph, I always recommend vitamins that are well rounded and complete as close to Mother Nature, as in fruits and vegetables and other foods. I recommend taking both vitamin D2 and D3. If you cannot find the combination I have made it into one capsule, and it is vegetarian. You can contact us at www.agingalternative.com or call 631-361-6160.

Typically, only a vitamin D 25 level is performed. One should also get a vitamin D 1-25 level. If the 1-25 D form is on high side or above normal with a slightly low vitamin D 25, I would not supplement unless you have cancer or an autoimmune disease. I have found people with this profile have vascular calcifications! I am writing a paper on this situation. If you have this profile I would also get an carotid artery doppler and cardiac CT scan for calcium score to see if you are coating your arteries and possible the valves of your heart with calcium!

Recently, vitamin D has been shown to have several applications. For several years it has been known that it is needed for bone density. Then it was noted that people who had low levels of (or a deficiency in) of vitamin D had an increase in cancer. Approximately a year ago from this writing, it was discovered that people with low levels also had increased cardiovascular and collagen vascular disease. However, one shouldn't blindly take vitamin D without getting a blood test to see if they actually need to supplement.

Vitamin D, as with other fat-soluble vitamins (A, E, K), is not without side effects. Fat-soluble vitamins are stored in the liver, and if large amounts are taken, they can build up and become toxic and cause side effects. For me, troubling side effects include calcification of blood vessels and soft tissue, as with Mr. Juda's case discussed above. Other possible side effects are hypercalemia (high calcium), hypercalcuria (calcium in the urine), nephrotoxicity (kidney damage), hyperphosphatemia (high phosphate), a dynamic bone disease (deficiencies in laying down bone), nausea, vomiting, anemia, weakness, and renal impairment. These side effects are usually seen with high-dose replacement of fifty thousand units or more per day.

It was a no-brainer to me approximately twenty-five years ago that high-dose vitamin Bs taken for extended periods of time could increase the incidence of cancer. Several of the vitamin Bs are required for DNA replication; therefore, if one takes high doses for a prolonged period of time, this could drive cells to replicate uncontrollably, which is what occurs in cancer cells.

This has unfortunately been proven medically true. For more details, see p. 95 in *Cancer Principles & Practice of Oncology Review,* second edition, or the textbook titled *Cancer* by DeVita, Hellman, and Rosenberg. You can also Google "vitamins causing cancer" and find other of medical references.

A good thing came out of the observation that vitamin Bs can cause cancer. Several drugs have been designed that block the function of vitamin Bs. An example of this is two drugs commonly used for cancer: methotrexate and pemetrexed. Both block folate (one form of vitamin B).

Therefore, baseline blood tests are needed to establish the deficiency or suboptimal level. If replacement with supplements is given, a repeat level should be obtained to ensure that a safe normal level is obtained. *Too much can be as bad as or sometimes worse than too little! This is a very important concept to remember.*

There are many potential chemotherapy, radiation, herbal, and supplement interactions. If you have a cancer and are being treated with chemotherapy and want to utilize supplements and herbals, you should see a physician well versed in both, for the best results. If not utilized correctly, they can work against each other and decrease effectiveness of the chemotherapy or cause additional side effects.

I must also caution you that even if the appropriate supplements are prescribed, they are sometimes mixed with ingredients you would not want in your body. I was recently reading the label on a box of vitamins that had a combination of calcium and vitamin D. It looked to be a good product, but on further reading I noted that aluminum was added! So while you were presumably taking a "good" supplement, you were also ingesting a toxic heavy metal, substituting one problem for another.

I recently had a male patient with a mildly high aluminum level and a true symptomatic testosterone deficiency. He was started on testosterone patches to be applied to the skin. Subsequent blood tests revealed the aluminum level to be mysteriously rising. I called the company that made the patches, and to my surprise these patches, which absorb into the skin, were made with aluminum.

Vegetarians may need to take supplements to compensate for what they are lacking in their diets. Many supplements, such as gel caps, are likely made, using animal products (gelatin capsules are made from hooves and hair of animals). There are product lines that are vegetarian friendly. Gary Null sells foods and supplements, books, DVDs, and other products for vegetarians through his website (see the references section at the end of this book).

Another word of caution to people who try to live healthy, including vegetarians: *no one is immune to disease, including cancers! Steve Jobs and Linda McCartney were both educated, well-to-do financially, and vegetarians, and both died from cancer.*

In summation there are vast arrays of conventional medications and supplements that are used to promote health and well-being. When any of these are used, it is essential to be an "educated consumer." You must research and understand the individual medicines and supplements that you take and any potential interactions between them. Again, your physician is your best resource, but you have to be your own health advocate.

CHAPTER 11
MISGUIDED DECISIONS

THE BODYBUILDER

A forty-two-year-old female came to me for advice regarding her bodybuilding career. She had been bodybuilding for approximately twenty years. She primarily worked out to look and feel young. She also competed in some bodybuilding contests. She worked out religiously six to seven days a week.

She was very critical of how she looked to the point that it had become obsessive and dangerous to her health. The term used for such an obsession for one's looks is called *body dysmorphic disorder*. She was taking extremely high doses of a strong prescription diuretic called Lasix. The doses were more than ten times as high as I and several other doctors have ever prescribed for even end-stage heart-disease patients.

She was also taking thyroid medication. This was not based on blood tests indicating low thyroid hormone. She would also take "speed" before contests to "cut up." She ate excessive amounts of meat to "build my muscles." She drank only one to two glasses of water a day in order to "not be bloated."

Her blood tests showed that she was causing kidney damage. In spite of this it took well more than a year for her to quit taking the medications that had not been prescribed by a physician. She was physically and psychologically dependent, which made it difficult to stop the medications, eat less meat, and drink more water.

After three to four months of correcting the above and taking supplements, her kidney function returned to normal. Now approximately two years afterward, her kidney function remains normal.

I have treated another patient for self-induced kidney problems. He would not stop eating excessive amounts of protein in order to maintain his massive muscularity. He was a very nice person but did not take heed and eventually required a kidney transplant.

THE DEATH OF A MOM

A thirty-four-year-old mother of two discovered a lump in her right breast. She thought it was a cyst. She applied "warm herbal soaks" for approximately three months. The lump enlarged, and the skin dimpled inward. She went to her doctor, who recommended a biopsy. She refused and continued to do "natural things."

She consulted with me approximately eleven months afterward. The lump was now the size of a lemon, and foul-smelling fluid was oozing out! She still thought it wasn't cancer and surgery was not needed. Her family and I begged her to reconsider. Finally she agreed to have a biopsy and full work-up.

Of course it was cancer, but it had traveled to her brain. She had chemotherapy and radiation, but the cancer took her over and she passed on. I will never forget her two young daughters running around the chemotherapy room and playing!

At the risk of being redundant, I will repeat: *If it is cancer, remove it as soon as possible!* Don't wait till it festers and travels to other areas of your body! Remove it early and you'll have a chance to be cured!

Benjamin Franklin said, "The man who does things makes mistakes, but he never makes the biggest mistake of all: doing nothing."

My Grandfather

My grandfather would sweat profusely for no apparent reason. He did not go to a doctor! What he did was take his friend's "heart pill." He had no clue as to why he was sweating or what the medicine was or its possible side effects. This case is a no-brainer but must be discussed. Frequently people do not go to the appropriate health-care provider when necessary.

Many years after, when my grandfather's legs filled with water, he went to a doctor. He was found to have severe aortic stenosis. This was causing all of his symptoms for all those years! Due to his age and the heart damage that was done from the longstanding aortic stenosis, artificial valve surgery was not done. He passed approximately a year later. Why this happened is quite amazing to me, but it was what I call *innocent ignorance.* If he would have taken care of this sooner, he might have lived much longer.

This also applies to vitamin supplements. You should not blindly take supplements. Just because it's labeled "natural" or "organic" or is an herbal product doesn't mean it's safe and/ or the correct dose for you. Blood tests are available for most vitamins. Remember, *too much of something including vitamins can be as bad as too little!* Too little vitamin D can cause vascular calcification, as does an excessive amount. You should get a blood test that includes vitamin levels.

I have cared for patients who experienced chest pain but did not immediately seek medical attention. This can be very dangerous and can cause heart damage and even death. No one is immune, even people who take supplements, exercise, and are vegetarian. When you think there might be something wrong, don't bury your head in the sand because you might bury the rest of your body with it! It has been said, "It is what it feels like."

LIMITATIONS OF DIAGNOSTIC TESTS

A relative of mine was experiencing chest pain. He went to a cardiologist for an evaluation. He was examined and an EKG was read as normal. No further tests were performed, and he was diagnosed as having muscular chest pain. No medications were prescribed.

A year went by and he still was experiencing chest discomfort. I called the cardiologist and begged for a stress thallium to be performed. One week afterward it was performed and read as negative.

The pain continued, even while at rest. Since stress thallium testing is approximately 85 percent sensitive, 15 percent of patients could have heart disease that could be missed. I discussed this with the cardiologist. A cardiac cauterization was performed and interpreted as positive! Sometimes you have to push your doctor and/or the system to get answers. You have to be your own health advocate! Sometimes to get what you want, you have to be pleasantly persistent and agreeably aggressive!

The Patient Knows Best

A wife of a doctor I worked with had recurrent pancreatitis. She was a vegan, took supplements, and exercised regularly. She lived in Manhattan and went to several highly recommended specialists. Several blood tests and scans were performed. She was told, "We don't know why you're having pancreatitis; all the tests are negative." She insisted that there *had to be a reason* for her recurrent pancreatitis.

She came to me for further testing. We performed several tests that had not been done before. We found her to have too much iron in her body. This is called *hemochromatosis* (iron overload). This condition can cause many health problems, including pancreatitis, heart disease, and liver cancer. She has been getting phlebotomized to remove the excessive iron. She has not had another attack of pancreatitis since!

Point is, if you think something is wrong, don't be satisfied without an answer! Remember, the squeaky wheel gets oiled. At the risk of being redundant: you have to be your own health advocate. If your family doctor and/or specialist can't find the answer, go to an alternative physician. Of course if your alternative clinician can't find the answer, whether the diagnoses or the treatment, go to your physician.

CHAPTER 12

FREQUENTLY ASKED QUESTIONS

The first question that is asked of my secretary when a prospective patient calls is whether I am an MD. First, it has been sometimes said in the realm of alternative medicine that many practitioners are not MDs/DOs (doctor of osteopathy), and many well-known, published people who are considered experts have had no formal medical training. There are alternative practitioners who are MDs, many of them specialists in other fields, who have not spent their lives studying alternative medicine and applying its principles.

Some patients have expressed that their alternative physician told them they decided at some point in their studies that they wished to pick an "easier" course, with no nights spent on-call in a hospital. This attempt to simplify happens in many businesses, professions, and with mainstream doctors. Like a businessman would approach an untapped market, clinicians perceive antiaging and complementary medicine as a new, yet-untapped field they wish to capitalize on.

However, there are knowledgeable and sincere individuals who care for patients. They may not be physicians, or are physicians with no formal training in these specialties. You as the patient should select a physician or other health-care practitioner you feel comfortable with in all regards. There are organizations in the references section that can assist you in this.

Recently, a physician I have known for years came to see me as a patient. I performed my usual new-patient exam. To my surprise, at the conclusion of the visit, he informed me he had only come in to learn how I ran my practice and see which tests I ordered on my patients so he could "do the same." This disheartened me because he wanted to practice without any true understanding, experience, or training in this type of medicine.

So how does one find a doctor well versed and experienced in alternative and antiaging medicine? The simplest way is to ask your doctor whether he or she can recommend anyone. While at the beginning of my practice several years ago, I felt resentment from some practitioners who did not know much about this field, I am happy to say now that I receive many referrals from colleagues, and together we work synergistically towards the goal of improved patient care. I am a board-certified oncologist, yet other oncologists send patients to me who are on chemotherapy and radiation treatments because I have a balanced approach, and I can enhance the response of their treatment and help buffer the side effects with supplements, nutrition, and many other alternative therapies.

If your physician does not know an alternative or antiaging physician, there are many organizations that can be helpful in locating a physician, such as the American Board of Holistic and Integrative Medicine; the American Board of Anti-Aging Medicine; the American Board of Integrative and Complementary Medicine; and the American Board of Nutrition. See the reference section or call my office at 631-361-6160 for further information.

CHAPTER 13
REASONS PEOPLE MAKE DEADLY TREATMENT MISTAKES

Why do people *incorrectly* utilize alternative and traditional treatments? They strive to use the most effective methods for the best possible quality of life and survival benefit but often fall short. There are several common reasons that cause this—I've seen this cost several patients their lives! This includes but is not limited to denial (which can be willful or what I call optimistic), benign neglect, procrastination, misinformation, fear (over concerns of appearance and other side effects of treatment), and the "I can outsmart it" syndrome.

Benign neglect is a patient who just doesn't think whatever he or she has is of any significance and doesn't react as most would to the given situation. The patient ignores what most would react to. This reaction could be due to lack of knowledge and to upbringing.

Denial can cause a patient to delay curative treatment to the point that it is no longer curable! Denial can be defined as a coping and defense mechanism. It is a primitive defense mechanism used by children to protect their ego from extreme anxiety in the midst of a dark and painful external reality.

There can be different degrees of denial. The first degree of denial is "I don't have it." Typically, a patient may have a breast lump, high blood pressure, elevated cholesterol, or high blood sugar and does not seek medical attention—or does but then doesn't follow up with recommendations.

The second degree of denial is "I know I have it, but I can beat it my way." I call this *optimistic denial.* A patient may have a deadly cancer that may be curable with conventional therapy. Examples of highly curable cancers are testicular carcinoma, Hodgkin's lymphoma, non-Hodgkin's lymphoma, and some early prostate and breast cancers. *To delay surgical removal of a localized cancer could cost a patient his or her life.* I have seen many patients die needlessly because they did not immediately remove the cancer.

To delay chemotherapy and radiation in cases of testicular, Hodgkin's lymphoma, non-Hodgkin's lymphoma, and other cancers could also be fatal. Along with these therapies, alternative treatments should be added to enhance the cure rate and decrease side effects.

You have to kill it before it kills you!

Some patients know they have a deadly cancer but delay treatment. They have many excuses that do not make logical sense. A commonly excuse is "I have no time right now." My response to that is "If you die from the cancer you definitely will have no time." They also frequently rationalize their situation by thinking, *It can't be cancer, I feel too well,* or *I feel well so I want to wait a while before I do anything.*

Occasionally a patient who has a localized tumor will be scheduled to have surgery in two months. This in my mind is procrastination on the side of medical care being given. It only takes a few cells to travel to other areas of the body and create a much worse disease and lessen the patient's chance of survival!

Take charge of your health and be pleasantly persistent and agreeably aggressive, but get the surgery done sooner.

Misinformation is another cause of needless pain, suffering, and death. There are people and many products that claim in one manner or another to be effective in treating heart disease, cancer, diabetes, hypertension, and other diseases that can be life threatening. But these products are not proven, or have been debunked and do not make any medical sense as to why they might be possibly effective.

Some patients want to "do it totally natural." I understand this and live naturally, but sometimes this will not yield the best results. Sometimes your body is not "a good friend," as Cat Stevens said in one of his songs. It is natural for the body to age and die. As we age, it appears that some become more prone to illness and overt diseases. This is natural, but I don't want any of it. Do you?

If you have a serious illness, don't look at it through foggy lenses. Do not let your illness become disgustingly clear and take you over. If you have cancer or end-stage heart disease, you are dealing with a monster that is in you, and it needs to be killed.

On the flipside of the coin, some patients say they were told all they need is chemotherapy and to "forget all the rest." I believe one should use all possible therapies in a manner that they complement rather than interfere with one another. As one patient said, "Doc, I want to kick, punch, strangle, radiate, poison, drown, shoot, and cut my cancer out."

Don't get stuck on one method of treatment. You are dealing with the demon within you that wants to kill you! Cancer is the ultimate suicide bomber. It kills you, the host, and it therefore dies!

When dealing with a deadly cancer, severe end-stage heart disease, diabetes, or hypertension, you cannot assume an alternative treatment will be totally effective and use it exclusively without medical guidance. You should consult a doctor who knows and utilizes both alternative and traditional approaches. This will enable you to make the best quality of life and optimal survival decisions in a safe fashion. Don't let misinformation cause you to make misguided decisions.

Regarding cancer and severe heart disease, some patients do not correctly connect the dots. They simply don't get the fact that if they don't do certain treatments in a rapid fashion, they could drastically reduce their chance of survival and/or cure and die needlessly.

Some patients dwell on the possible side effects of treatment and not on the fact that the disease will kill them if not treated. Sometimes you need real soldiers and not toy ones to get the job done. You are not a superhero and immune to the possible consequences!

You should be aware of the possible side effects, but take advantage of the benefits!

In the face of an acute heart attack, you may need an emergency coronary artery stent surgically placed, or may even need a bypass. Acute leukemias, aggressive lymphomas, other cancers, severe allergic reactions, acute asthmatic attack, and other medical situations may require immediate "strong guns" with no-holds-barred treatments for the best survival outcome. There may simply be no time to try anything else. These medical situations need to be treated rapidly and definitively or you may suffer needlessly or potentially die.

Some patients are concerned with the possibility of cancer cells leaching out and being spread through aspiration or fine-needle biopsy procedures. Some doctors don't think this is a major concern. I, however, have some concerns that it could possibly cause some cells to be mobilized and spread.

Furthermore, some feel the correct diagnosis can be missed when using such procedures. In other words, the biopsy or aspiration done was not of the cancerous area of tumor, so it read as negative for cancer. Time passes, and the lump in the breast grows and the repeat biopsy is positive for cancer. As a result, the cancer is at a more advanced stage requiring even more aggressive surgery, radiation, and chemotherapy.

The book *Hematology and Oncology Subspecialty Consult*, second edition, by the Department of Medicine, University School of Medicine, on p. 192, regarding breast cancer, states, "Excisional biopsy is the gold standard, allowing complete histological characterization with regard to biomarkers as well as tumor grade. Excisional biopsy also may serve as the definitive lumpectomy."

Whenever possible, get an excisional biopsy to remove the entire tumor! This will enable the pathologist to look at the entire tumor and avoid making an inadvertent misdiagnosis. This will avoid possible cancer cells from spreading from the surgical procedure. Also, the suspicious lump will have been removed, and therefore future worry and concern about it.

Some patients are so fearful, they don't take action for too long a period. The saying "the best defense is a good offense" is applicable to preventing and treating disease and fighting the aging process.

Others focus on only the negatives of treatment. Of course the benefits of treatment should outweigh the possible side effects. Treatment decisions can be difficult at times. Again, you should consult with a physician who is complementary/integrative in his approach. Usually four eyes see better than two, and two heads are better than one!

I have had patients who delayed their treatment because they were afraid of losing their hair. You can grow your hair back, not your life!

Some patients are afraid of surgery causing disfigurement. Cosmetic surgery has come a long way, and disfigurement is minimal. Don't delay your treatment and let your cancer grow and travel to other organs and reduce your chances of possible cure!

Don't fear tomorrow. You can be there if you go forward and take the appropriate steps.

On the other side of cosmetics we have the opposite situation, where someone takes drugs to get a particular advantage in an unsafe manner. This was discussed earlier regarding the bodybuilder and the patient with mild acne. Our society has become overmedicated in some instances. Bodybuilders have an expression, "Medication for dedication." This is not the truth. I have been exercising regularly for forty-five years without such assistance.

The balance is obvious to most, but not all, which is to take medication only when absolutely necessary. Always weigh the benefit-versus-side-effect profile. Indeed, medications can be lifesaving and necessary.

A catchy drug commercial I heard spun words very well in favor of taking a drug. It said to "be aware of the possible side effects and take advantage of the benefits." Be an educated consumer at all times. If it is a tough, not black-or-white, decision, consult an appropriate specialist for advice. You have to make the ultimate decision.

Some patients distrust conventional medicine, which causes them not to utilize effective treatments. I have heard patients say that "doctors don't want cures because they would go out of business." This is simply not true. I feel ridiculous even entertaining this, but if there was a cure for a disease, the doctor would have to see the patient, make a diagnosis, treat, and appropriately follow up. He would still have a job!

It has also been said that drug companies don't want cures. I hope this is not true! I do have many bones to pick with drug companies, but I think if there was a major breakthrough, as there have been, they would capitalize on it and make a lot of money. Therefore, they would not hold back on cures and other breakthroughs. This is one major way they make money.

Delay of treatment can be also caused by truly difficult situations. In some cases, minor delays might be actually advantageous. Sometimes diagnoses and treatment choices are very gray. This is especially true when dealing with cancer. A typical example of this situation is breast cancer. A test called an "oncotype" tells a patient the percentage chance of her breast cancer returning after it is removed. Some feel that the oncotype test is not very accurate. Some feel it does not take into consideration all related factors. That is another argument, but be that as it may, it is used by oncologists.

Here is a typical quagmire when using the oncotype test. It causes distress to the well-read breast cancer patient. An example of a difficult decision via the oncotype is when it states that you have a 20 percent chance of the breast cancer returning, that if you take conventional chemotherapy, it will reduce this to 11 percent.

The patient then Googles the drugs that are going to be used and notes that they can cause secondary cancers and other possible major side effects! Again you should go to an oncologist you are comfortable with and make an educated decision. It is your personal decision.

"The gambler" is a patient who knows he has a deadly disease but chooses to "take a chance." He is typically a male with a dominant and opinionated personality. When dealing with cancer or heart disease, it's not the time to roll the dice. You will lose big-time! The odds are against you. You have to shuffle the cards and deal with it. Don't chase a dream that won't come true.

There is a Yiddish saying: "Ten enemies cannot hurt a man as much as he hurts himself." Don't hurt yourself!

CHAPTER 14

SUMMARY

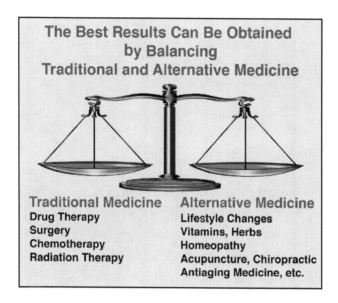

The Best Results Can Be Obtained
by Balancing
Traditional and Alternative Medicine

Traditional Medicine
Drug Therapy
Surgery
Chemotherapy
Radiation Therapy

Alternative Medicine
Lifestyle Changes
Vitamins, Herbs
Homeopathy
Acupuncture, Chiropractic
Antiaging Medicine, etc.

It is my hope that this book has pointed out the differences and similarities between conventional and alternative medicines, and how they can complement each other to treat disease and prolong health and life span. Clearly, the rationale and the treatment modalities are often conflicting and oppositional. What is more important than the differences are the many similarities, such as agreement about the importance of prevention, exercise, nutrition, rest, sleep, vitamins, and risk factor modifications (e.g., stopping smoking, consuming moderate levels of alcohol, and eliminating obesity).

What has guided me throughout my medical career is the realization that there does not have to be a choice as to which approach to take. Medical care and treatment should be a *balance* of these two approaches. They should work synergistically and in harmony to increase health span and life span. Even in patients with severe illnesses, an alternative practitioner can improve their general nutritional status and well-being, enhance immune responses, and offer supplements to enhance the positive effects of medication, radiation, surgery, and chemotherapy.

There may be of course a situation where a patient will have to make a decision between standard medical and alternative/natural treatment. The decision should be an educated one based on the track record of each treatment modality. The effectiveness and short- and long-term side effects and benefits should be investigated. One should weigh all arguments, pros and cons. The decision shouldn't be rushed. In carpentry, there is a well-known expression: "Measure twice and cut once."

Integrative medicine not only emphasizes the physician-patient relationship, it focuses on the least invasive, least toxic methods to promote health by integrating allopathic and alternative therapies. Remember, you and your physician are partners in your health care. There should be trust in your physician and a relationship that is comfortable enough for you to ask questions about your health and treatment.

In my practice, my consultations are detailed and extensive, intending to get to the medical root of the problem while determining the patient's health care goals. Then, an individualized prescription for care is determined with the patient's active involvement in formulating this plan. Over time, goals and plans change based on clinical response. As previously stated, health care is dynamic, not static.

Remember:

- Combine standard and alternative therapeutics in a logically balanced, safe, and scientific fashion. This can prevent disease and extend health and life span. This will also increase longevity and a sense of well-being and decrease side effects of treatments and reoccurrence of an existing disease.

- You have to be your own health advocate; however, *a person with good judgment does not rely solely on himself!* In fact it has been said that a doctor who takes care of himself has a fool for a patient, and a doctor who is committing malpractice! Find a physician who balances Eastern and Western medical practices and work with him or her. If you cannot, please feel free to call my Long Island office at 631-361-6160.

- There is a *fine line between hype and hope*. It is easy to believe something is effective if you want it to be so. You have to be objective! Do not rely on just what you feel or think may be happening. I call this mind-set "subjective truth." Don't get crippled by dogma.

- If you are not getting the desired results, *don't keep doing what you have been doing. You'll only get what you've gotten.* Insanity according to Albert Einstein is "doing the same thing over and over again and expecting different results." Try different approaches under the guidance of your health-care practitioner.

- Too much of a supplement, vitamin, herb, or medicine can be as bad as or even worse than too little. Vitamin D deficiency and excess can both cause vascular calcifications. I have been testing and treating vitamin D deficiencies for many years. The importance of vitamin D has finally been recognized by mainstream medicine. A deficiency is usually treated with fifty thousand units of vitamin D2 (D2 is synthetic and manufactured and is handled via prescription while D3 is a natural version that you can buy over-the-counter) one to two times a week. I consider D3 an industrial-strength treatment for most patients because the usual dosage of vitamin D3 is less than ten thousand units, and the RDA is as low as a thousand units, which is really just too low to be of any benefit. I feel this megadose (fifty thousand units) approach is often appropriate for severe vitamin D deficiencies and for cancer patients.

- Get vitamin blood levels checked before you take anything in a high dose. If you are found to have a low level and are taking a replacement, you should periodically repeat the blood test to make sure you are taking the proper amount.

- Decrease your risks using preventative methods, including early detection (regular checkups, detailed blood tests, colonoscopies, body imaging studies, etc.).

- Eat raw, organic fruits and vegetables whenever possible.

- Drink at least eight glasses of high quality (filtered) water each day.

- Keep away from chemicals, additives, and other unnatural dangers (high-energy electrical devices, such as microwaves, hairdryers, electrical outlets by the head of the bed), heavy metals (e.g., cups, water bottles, pots, and pans, etc., made of aluminum).

- Have your home and workplace checked for radon, carbon monoxide, and air and water toxins.

- Use glass, stainless steel, or ceramic pots, pans, and glasses. Keep your own dishes and glasses at work. This is good for you and the environment. Styrofoam cups are bad for the environment and humans. This is especially true when Styrofoam cups and containers are microwaved, or hot and/ or acidic (coffee, tea) liquids are used in them. This causes the chemicals to leak out and be ingested. There are many chemicals in the Styrofoam and no one really knows what daily use of such cups and containers will do to the body over a prolonged period of time!

- Always be physically, intellectually, and socially active. Exercise regularly (aerobic, anaerobic, and mental activity).

- Maintain a positive attitude at all times.

- Have several goals whether they pertain to business, are physical or academic in nature, are pleasurable, or pertain to music, art, social activities, and/or are family-related. It has been said by many wise men and women that having *purpose* is essential for the well-being of an individual and our civilization as a whole.

- Make a plan, so when you're ready to pass on, you won't say to yourself, *I wish I would have done this or that!* Have a bucket list (things you want to do before you die). Make a plan detailing how and when you will do them and then do them!

- Don't postpone enjoyment!

- Regardless: "Don't compromise yourself. You are all you've got."—Janis Joplin

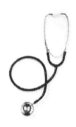 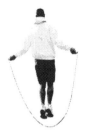 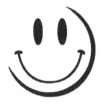

GOOD LUCK!

ABOUT THE AUTHOR

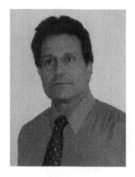 Richard Sollazzo, MD, has been following a healthy, natural lifestyle. He not only walks the walk, he sprints it! He has attempted to pass on some of his methodology to others, first as a naturopath and chiropractor, and later as a physician for the past twenty-five years. He humbly believes you never graduate from the "university of learning." As a result he has devoted his life to learning. He has become board certified in internal medicine, oncology, hematology, geriatrics, sports medicine, emergency medicine, antiaging, complementary/integrative medicine, holistic medicine, and nutrition. In 2003, he formally created a complementary/integrative medical practice called Aging Alternatives, with offices located in Manhattan and on Smithtown, Long Island.

He has his own cable TV public-service show, *Shock the World with Health and Goodness.* He has also appeared multiple times on TV with alternative practitioner Dr. Gary Null. He has written for numerous local papers and magazines on various topics in medicine, has given health lectures to the community, and has provided information and blogs covering antiaging and complementary medical topics on his website.

For more information on any of these topics, visit his website at www.AgingAlternative.com. If you have any questions and would like to speak to someone in Dr. Sollazzo's office, call 631-361-6160 (Long Island) or 212-935-1700 (Manhattan).

For continuing information, including blogs, video, and other media, please visit his website: www.AgingAlternative.com

Long Island office: 631-361-6160 (If you need to contact the doctor directly, this is the preferred office.)

Manhattan office: 212-935-1700

BIBLIOGRAPHY

Chapters 1 and 2:

None.

Chapter 3:

Eisenberg, David M., et al. "Unconventional Medicine in the United States: Prevalence, Costs, and Pattern of Use." *New England Journal of Medicine* 328 (January 28, 1993): 246–52.

Prenguber, M. "Multidisciplinary Therapy: Integrated Medicine in Cancer Care." *American Journal of Hematology/Oncology*, October 2007.

Chapter 4:

None.

Chapter 5:

Brodov, Y., et al. "Usefulness of Combining Serum Uric Acid and C-Reactive Protein for Risk Stratification of Patients with

Coronary Artery Disease." *America Journal of Cardiology* 104 (July 15, 2009): 194–98.

Becker, et al. "Simvastatin versus Therapeutic Lifestyle Changes and Supplements: Randomized Primary Prevention Trial." *Mayo Clinic Proceedings* 83, no. 7 (July 2008): 758–63.

Halbert, Steven C., et al. "Tolerability of Red Yeast Rice (2,400 mg Twice Daily) versus Pravastatin (20 mg Twice Daily) in Patients with Previous Statin Intolerance." *American Journal of Cardiology* 105, no. 2 (January 15, 2010): 198–204.

Holdaway, I. M. and H. G. Freisen. "Hormone Binding by Human Mammary Carcinoma." *Cancer Research* 37 (1977): 1946–52.

Ornish, Dean, MD, et al. "Can Lifestyle Changes Reverse Coronary Heart Disease? The Lifestyle Heart Trial." *The Lancet* 336 (1990): 129–33.

Miller, Edgar R., et al. "Meta-Analysis: High-Dosage Vitamin E Supplementation May Increase All-Cause Mortality." *Annals of Internal Medicine 142*, no. 1 (January 4, 2005): 37–46.

Stampfer, M., et al. Nurses' Health Study, 328 (1993): 1444.

Stechschulte, S. A., et al. "Vitamin D: Bone and Beyond: Rationale and Recommendations for Supplementation." *American Journal of Medicine* 122, no. 9 (September 2009): 793–802.

Stevens, N. G., et al. "Randomized Controlled Trial of Vitamin E in Patients with Coronary Disease: Cambridge Heart Antioxidant Study (CHAO S)." *The Lancet* 23, no. 347 (March 1996): 781–86.

Chapter 6:

European Journal of Oncology 17 (1981): 1223–28) article by Alabaster, O., it stated that metabolic modification by insulin enhances methotrexate (a commonly used chemotherapeutic agent) cytotoxicity in MCF-7 human breast cancer cells. It was also stated that *insulin utilized with methotrexate could possibly increase ten-thousand-fold the cytotoxic effect!*

Pavelic, K. "Correlation of Substances Immunologically Cross-Reactive with Insulin, Glucose, and Growth Hormone in Hodgkin's Lymphoma Patients." *Cancer Letters* 17 (1982): 81–6.

Schilsky, R. "Characteristics of Membrane Transport of Methotrexate by Cultured Human Breast Cancer Cells." *Biochemistry Pharmacology* 30 (1981): 1537–42.

Gross, G. "Pertubalation by Insulin of Human Breast Cancer Cell Kinetics." *Cancer Research* 44 (1984): 3570–75.

Link, J., MD. *The Breast Survival Cancer Manual.* 5th ed. New York: Holt Paperbacks, 2012.

Hauser, Ross A. and Marion A. Hauser. *Treating Cancer with Insulin Potentiation Therapy*. Oak Park, Ill.: Beulah Land Press, 2002.

Kushi, M. *The Cancer Prevention Diet, Revised and Updated Edition: The Macrobiotic Approach to Preventing and Relieving Cancer*. New York: St. Martin's Griffin, 2009.

Servan-Schreiber, D. Anticancer: *A New Way of Life, New Edition*. New York: Viking, 2009.

Ayre, Steven G., et al. *The Kinder, Gentler Cancer Treatment: Insulin Potentiation Targeted LowDose™ Therapy*. Charleston, S. C.: BookSurge Publishing, 2009.

Moss, Ralph W. *Questioning Chemotherapy*. Equinox Press, 1995.

Chapter 7:

Hall, Susan A., et al. "Sexual Activity, Erectile Dysfunction, and Incident Cardiovascular Events." *The American Journal of Cardiology* 105, no. 2 (January 15, 2010): 192–97.

Life Extension Organization publishes a monthly magazine containing articles on alternative and antiaging medicine. Also see their book *Disease Prevention and Treatment*, which contains a wealth of information. www.lef.org.

Groopman, Jerome. *How Doctors Think*. Reprint ed. Boston: Mariner Books, 2008.

Klatz, R., and Robert Goldman. *7 Anti-aging Secrets for Optimal Digestion and Scientific Weight Loss*. Elite Sports Medicine Publications, 1996.

McGully, Kilmer S. *The Homocysteine Revolution*. New York: McGraw-Hill, 1999.

Morley, J., and Lucretia van den Berg. *Endocrinology of Aging (Contemporary Endocrinology)*. Totowa, N.J. Humana Press, 1999.

Park, Alice. "The Science of Living Longer: How to Live 100 Years." *TIME* 175, no. 7 (February 22, 2010).

Pearson, D., and Sandy Shaw. *Life Extension: A Practical Scientific Approach*. New York: Warner Books, 1983.

Shippen, E., and William Fryer. *The Testosterone Syndrome: The Critical Factor for Energy, Health, and Sexuality—Reversing the Male Menopause*. M. Evans and Company, Inc., 2001.

Warren, Michelle P. and Naama W. Constantini. *Sports Endocrinology (Contemporary Endocrinology)*. Totowa, N.J. Humana Press, 2010.

Smith, Roy G., and Michael O. Thorner, eds. *Human Growth Hormone: Research and Clinical Practice (Contemporary endocrinology)*. Totowa, N.J. Humana Press, 2000.

Chapter 8:

Clinical Update, *Emergency Medicine* (August 2003): 33–36.

Jovanovic-Peterson, L., and S. Levert. *A Woman Doctor's Guide to Menopause: Essential Facts and Up-To-The-Minute Information for a Woman's Change of Life.* New York: Hyperion, 1993.

IMPORTANT WEBSITES AND REFERENCES

ACUPUNCTURE AND HERBAL THERAPIES

* Jordan Barber MS, Lac, LMT. Licensed acupuncturist, massage therapist, and Rife therapist. For blogs and latest research, visit his website at www.Sirius-Wellness.com.

* Kelly Ann Parish MS, LAc, LMT. Licensed acupuncturist and massage therapist. Applied kinesiology, bio-energetic testing, NAET certified practitioner at Sirius Wellness. www.Sirius-Wellness.com.

ADDICTION WEBSITES

Alcohol Abuse

* www.aaa.com.

* www.SoberRecovery.com.

* www.BottleBlocker.info—For info on deterring teen drinking using a tamper-proof locking device.

Alcohol, Natural Treatments

- www.habitdoc.com.

- www.BottleBlocker.info—For info on deterring teen drinking using a tamper-proof locking device.

Drugs

- www.drug-addiction.com.

- www.drugabuse.gov/PODAT

- www.BottleBlocker.info—For info on deterring teen RX drug abuse at home.

Smoking Cessation

- www.quit-smoking.com.

- www.webmd.com/smoking-cessation.

- Carr, Allen. *The Easy Way to Stop Smoking: Join the Millions Who Have Become Non-Smokers Using Allen Carr's EasyWay Method.* New York: Sterling, 2010.

ALTERNATIVE MEDICINE

Antiaging

- www.agingalternative.com.

- Gary Null, PhD: www.garynull.com.

  800-562-0523

  Dr. Null is a leading alternative health and nutrition expert. He has written many books about natural living and healing. He is an award-winning talk radio host and natural healing advocate. He has created many excellent TV shows, DVDs, and CDs.

  He is an advocate for freedom of health choices. Books he has written on this subject include *The Complete Encyclopedia of Natural Healing*, *The Complete Guide to Health and Nutrition*, and *The Clinician's Handbook of Natural Healing*.

- National Institutes for Health National and Center for Complementary and Alternative Medicine: http://nccam. nih.gov/health.

- New York Online Access to Health Directory of Websites and Resources: www.noah-health.org/en/alternative/ty.

- McMaster University Health Care Information Resources Alternative Medicine Directory of Websites: http://hsl.lib. mcmaster.ca/tomflem/almed.html.

- Kids' health website on complementary and alternative medicine for teens: www.kidshealth.org/teen/your_body/medical_care/alternative_medicine.html.

- American Society of Anesthesiologists—Information on dietary supplements when preparing for surgery: www.asahq.org/patientEducation/herbpatient.pdf.

- Alternative Medicine Foundation: Nonprofit education, information organization about the integration of alternative and conventional medicine for public and professionals: www.amfoundation.org/faqs.htm.

- The American College of Physicians (ACP): *Guide to Complementary & Alternative Medicine*, published in 2009. More information from the ACP is available at: www.acponline.org/acp_press/comp_alt_med.

- Jonas, Wayne B., ed. *Mosby's Dictionary of Complementary & Alternative Medicine*, New York: Elsevier, 2004.

ANTIAGING AND RELATED TOPICS

- www.agingalternative.com.

- www.optimalagingsolutions.com.

- The American Academy of Anti-Aging Medicine: www.worldhealth.net.

- www.garynull.com.

- Life Extension Organization publishes a monthly magazine containing articles on alternative and antiaging medicine. Their book, *Disease Prevention and Treatment,* contains a wealth of information. www.lef.org.

- Groopman, J. *How Doctors Think.* Reprint ed. Boston: Mariner Books, 2008.

Cancer

- To learn more about insulin potentiation therapy (IPT), and other cancer therapies go to: www.AgingAlternatives.com.

- www.adjuvantoonline.com.

- www.breastlink.com.

- Life Extension Organization: www.lef.org.

- Caris Life Sciences test tumor samples for chemo sensitivity: www.carislifesciences.com.

Complementary and Alternative Medicine

- National Cancer Institute: www.cancer.gov.

- Gary Null, PhD: www.garynull.com.

- Life Extension Organization: www.lef.org.

- For a real eye-opener regarding many important health issues related to water, read F. Batmanghelidj's *Your Body's Many Cries for Water*. 3rd ed. Global Health Solutions, Inc., 2008. www.watercure.com.

- Jonas, Wayne B., ed. *Mosby's Dictionary of Complementary & Alternative Medicine*, New York: Elsevier, 2004.

- Luanne Pennesi, RN, MS, is a well-known consultant who deals with lifestyle in a detailed fashion. She has helped many patients optimize their health and worked with those with overt diseases. Visit her website: www.metropolitanwellness.com.

COSMETICS

- For information on many consumer products including cosmetics that can contain toxic chemicals and heavy metals: www.ewg.org.

- Hair transplants: world-renowned specialist Robert Dorin, DO, diplomat of the American Board Hair Restoration Surgery. Visit www.truedorin.com or call 212-826-2525.

ENERGY MEDICINE

- For more information on ozone therapy, hyperbaric therapy, and oxidative therapy, visit the American College for Advancement in Medicine's website, www.acam.org.

ENVIRONMENTAL AND OTHER HAZARDOUS EXPOSURES

- www.Healthyhomeinspectioninc.com or call 631-672-9768 This company provides in home assessments of environmental hazards and cancer risk.

- www.BottleBlocker.info—For info on deterring toddlers from gaining access to bottles with poisonous materials, using a tamper-proof locking device.

- www.AgingAlternative.com.

- Toxic release data by zip code: www.scorecard.org.

- Information on consumer products: cell phones, drinking water, vegetables and fruits (insecticides, pesticides), cosmetics, and other topics: www.ewg.org.

- For the latest info regarding environmental exposure: www.EnvironmentalhealthNews.org.

- Agency for Toxic Substances and Disease Registry: www.atsdr.cdc.gov/toxprofiles.

- The American College for Advancement in Medicine: Acam.org.

- Household product analysis: http://householdproducts.nih. gov/index.htm.

- Environmental Working Group (household and other products analysis): www.ewg.org.

- Maps, tables, text revealing geographic patterns of cancer death rates throughout the united states from 1950 to 1994 for approximately forty types of cancer. Cancer Mortality Maps & Graphs: www3.cancer.gov.

- Dadd, Debra Lynn. *The Nontoxic Home & Office.* New York, N.Y. Jeremy P. Tarcher, Inc., 1992.

EXERCISE

- Gary Null, PhD: Books he has written on this subject include *Ultimate Training: Gary's Null's Complete Guide to Eating Right, Exercise, and Living Longer;* and *Get Healthy Now! with Gary Null: A Complete Guide to Prevention, Treatment, and Healthy Living.* Visit www.garynull.com.

- Prevention magazine www.prevention.com.

GENERAL HEALTH

- Gary Null, PhD: www.garynull.com.

- *Prevention* magazine: www.prevention.com.

- Batmanghelidj, F. *Your Body's Many Cries for Water*. 3rd ed. Global Health Solutions, Inc., 2008. Falls Church , VA www.watercure.com.

HOLISTIC, INTEGRATIVE, AND COMPLEMENTARY MEDICINE

- www.AgingAlternative.com.

- American Board of Holistic Medicine: www.holisticboard.org.

- The American College for Advancement of Medicine provides training and certification in alternative medicine for physicians. Their emphasis is on chelation therapy and other IV treatments. Several seminars a year are given, and they publish several publications. Visit www.acam.org.

- The American Association of Integrative Medicine: www. aaimedicine.com.

- Groopman, J. *How Doctors Think*. Reprint ed. Boston: Mariner Books, 2008.

Hormones, Female/Male

- www.AgingAlternative.com.

- www.garynull.com.

- Suzanne Somers has written many books on health and hormone replacement. Her 2007 book *Ageless: The Naked Truth about Bioidentical Hormones* (Three Rivers Press) describes hormone replacement therapy for both men and women. Visit www.SuzanneSomers.com for more information.

- Life Extension Organization offers many articles on male andropause and female menopause and other hormonal issues. www.lef.org.

- Batmanghelidj, F. *Your Body's Many Cries for Water.* 3rd ed. Falls Church, VA. Global Health Solutions, Inc., 2008. www.watercure.com.

- This well-known book is considered one of the "bibles" of medicine. Kasper, Dennis L., et al. *Harrison's Manual of Medicine.* 16th ed. New York: McGraw Hill, 2005.

- http://www.mhprofessional.com/product.php?isbn=0071466983.

- Another well-known bible of medicine: *Cecil's Textbook of Medicine.* www.ceilmedicine.com.

- National Institutes of Health: www.nih.gov.

- National Comprehensive Cancer Network: www.nccn.org.

- Dr. Nick Delgado's article "Estrogen Dominance: A Newly Discovered Male Toxin" appeared in *Anti-Aging Medical News*. He has also published several other articles and books. His website is www.extendyouth.com.

- Vliet, Elizabeth L. *The Savvy Woman's Guide to Testosterone: How to Revitalize Your Sexuality, Strength and Stamina.* Tucson, AZ Press, 2005.

- Shippen, E. *The Testosterone Syndrome: The Critical Factor for Energy, Health, and Sexuality—Reversing the Male Menopause.* Tucson, AZ M. Evans and Company, Inc., 2001.

- Morley, J., and Lucretia van den Berg. *Endocrinology of Aging (Contemporary Endocrinology).* Totowa, N.J. Humana Press, 2011.

INSULIN POTENTIATION THERAPY (IPT)

- For more information about Insulin Potentiation Therapy, visit www.AgingAlternative.com or call 631-361-6160.

MUSCULOSKELETAL-RELATED INJURIES

- Manhattan Spine & Sports Therapy: www.manhattanspine. com. 212-935-1700. Specializing in physical therapy, chiropractic, ultrasound guided facet, nerve block, joint and trigger point injections. Epidural and joint rejuvenation platelet-rich plasma (PRP) and stem cell therapy as permitted.

OBESITY

- Gary Null, PhD: His titles include *Gary Null's Ultimate Lifetime Diet: A Revolutionary All-Natural Program for Losing Weight and Building a Healthy Body; Kiss Your Fat Goodbye: The Ultimate Guide to Losing Weight and Building a Healthy Body for Life;* and *The Vegetarian Handbook: Eating Right for Total Health.* Visit www.garynull.com.

- www.cdc.gov/obesity/index.html.

- www.obesity.org.

- www.agingalternitve.com.

- Child health/obesity: www.kidshealth.org.

- *Prevention* magazine: www.prevention.com.

Surgeons

- Richard Lazzaro M.D. Board Certified Thoracic Surgeon, pioneer in robotic surgery. (212) 434-4957—130-East 77th Street, N.Y., N.Y. 10075

Traditional Medicine

- www.AgingAlternative.com.

- Archives of Internal Medicine: www.archinternmed.com.

- National Institutes of Health: www.nih.gov.

- MedicineNet.com.

- Jacobs, Bradley P., and Katherine *Gundling. ACP Evidence-Based Guide to Complementary & Alternative Medicine.* The American College of Physicians, 2009.

- The America Journal of Cardiology: www.ajconline.org.

- National Cancer Institute: www.cancer.gov.

- National Comprehensive Cancer Network: www.nccn.org.

- The New England Journal of Medicine: www.nejm.org.

- The American Journal of Medicine: www.amjmed.com.

- PDR (Physicians Desk Reference) for herbal medicines, nutritional supplements, and drugs: www.pdr.net.

- WebMD: www.webmd.com.

- Journal of the American Medical Association: www.jama. ama-ass.org.

VEGETARIANISM

- Gary Null, PhD: www.garynull.com.